Gut Health

How to improve your Physical and mental well-being with a correct diet plan (leaky gut mental health anxiety)

Robert Francisco Diamond

are for clarifying purposes only and are the owned by the owners themselves, not affiliated with this document.

TABLE OF CONTENTS

INTRODUCTION

Chapter 1

INTESTINAL MICROCOSM

OUR (SECOND) BRAIN THAT WORKS BY BACTERIA

Chapter 2

WHERE DO OUR INTESTINAL BACTERIA COME FROM?

Chapter 3

THE LANGUAGE OF MICROBES: AN ESSENTIAL COMPONENT OF DIALOGUE BETWEEN INTESTINE AND BRAIN

Chapter 4

THE CONSEQUENCES OF AN UNBALANCED INTESTINAL MICROBIOTE ON OUR WELL-BEING

Chapter 5

CAUSES OF DYSBIOSIS INTESTINAL IATROGENE

Chapter 6

FEEDING BACTERIAL GROUP

Chapter 7

YOU ARE WHAT YOU EAT WHEN YOU TAKE ACCOUNT OF YOUR INTESTINAL MICROBES

Chapter 8

THE INTESTINAL MICROBIOTA AND OBESITY

Chapter 9

MICROBIOTA AND MENTAL WELL-BEING

Chapter 10

FATTY ACIDS THAT ACT AGAINST THE INFLAMMATORY STRESS

Chapter 11

RELEASE THE CHRONIC CONTRACTS THAT PREVENT VISCERAL EMOTIONS FROM BEING CARRIED OUT TO THE SURFACE, THE HARA MASSAGE

Chapter 12

WHAT WE CAN DO FOR THE HEALTH OF OUR MICROBIOME

Chapter 13

WHAT TO AVOID AND WHY, AND RECOMMENDATIONS

Chapter 14

FERMENTED DRINKS:

Chapter 15

MEDICINAL, EXTRACTED PLANTS, WHICH ARE CONSOLIDATED (AND TRADITIONAL) IN THE TREATMENT OF THE MAIN INTESTINAL INFLAMMATORY FORMS

Chapter 16

ESSENTIAL OILS

Conclusion

Introduction

The thing that always impressed me most in an anatomy lesson is the fact that we're only 10% human, and our microbes do the rest. I became curious to know more about these invisible creatures that keeps us alive. There was a moment, in my discovery of the microbes that inhabit the human body, in which I stopped considering myself as an individual and started to see myself as the container of my microbiota.

Now I consider myself and my microbiota as a team. Just like in any relationship, you only get what you give. I feed and protect them, and they also support and feed me in return. I find myself thinking about my food choices in terms of what my microbes would be grateful to receive, and my physical and mental health being an indicator of my ability to host them. They represent my colony, and their conservation has the same value for me as the well-being of the cells of my body.

Our intestine and its microcosm are a symbiosis that has a decisive influence on our health.

Two thousand five hundred years ago, Hippocrates, the father of modern medicine, believed that all diseases originated in the intestine.

He knew little about the anatomy of that organ, let alone the 100 trillion microbes that live there, but as we are learning two millennia later that he had made a significant discovery. Because the intestine is the only body organ that has a central nervous system that is capable of mediating reflexes in the complete absence of input from the brain or spinal cord. The intestine has long been considered as an unnecessary organ.

The surgeon of the King of England, Sir Arbuthnot Lane, hypothesized, about a hundred years ago, that the poisoning of our body originated from the large intestine. For this reason, it would have been advisable to remove it, even in the absence of disease. Fortunately, this vital organ has gained new importance with the affirmation of holistic medicine, thanks to the knowledge acquired by doctors and scientists, such as Ilya Metchnikoff or FX Mayr who stated that: "The intestine is for man what the root it's for the tree." Recent scientific studies confirm this theory.

During one of my walks in the woods, I thought about the root of the plants and how the small ends of these roots, microscopic root hairs extend into the soil to absorb the nutrients that microorganisms produce in the soil. And then I thought about the human intestine and how it is covered by microscopic villi, thin protuberances very similar to the root hairs, which point inside the intestine and absorb the nutrients from the digested elements of last night's dinner.

The intestine is like an upside down root; it carries the soil inside it; this is the adaptation that an eternity ago has used to distinguish animals from plants. It is as if the animals had learned to pull the roots out of the ground and turn them around so that they could move instead of sticking to a point.

Let us imagine a virgin rainforest, green and full of life, if a great diversity of species lives there, the living space is intact, and the soil is fertile. Now let's look at the woodcutters who arrives, destroys the forest that has been there for ages with a chainsaw (in the intestine the "deforestation" may correspond for example to antibiotic therapy or a monotonous diet). The forest will grow back in due time, but it will not be the same pristine, intricate, and intact habitat that it was before. There will be less diversity. The most sensitive species will not survive. The invaders will prosper. For the complex ecosystem of the intestine, on a scale of a million times smaller, the principle still holds.

Antibiotic chainsaws and invasive pathogens demolish the intertwining of life that has created a balance through infinite and subtle interactions. If the destruction has been sufficiently extended, the system fails to recover. On the contrary, it collapses. In the rainforest, this translates into habitat destruction. In the body, it causes dysbiosis or an anomaly in the balance of the microbiota. The ecosystem is intact only if composed of the most significant possible number of species. If harmony reigns in our microbiota, our health will also be excellent.

In the past, a sick intestine was distinguished from a healthy one by considering only the cells of the body and not the cells of the bacteria. Through billions of microorganisms, the intestine controls most of our body's metabolic processes, it produces vitamins, enzymes, and essential amino acids, as well as neutralizing all the toxic substances we put into our body through food.

If we dedicate a moment of attention to our intestinal mucosa, we will understand that we are relatively ignorant of our intestines. We easily perceive skin and muscles, even the mucous membranes of the nose and eyes, and with the tongue, we can explore the inside of the oral cavity.

We also perceive the morsel that slides into the esophagus, and perhaps we also realize when the stomach is full. But then the great unknown begins. The moment we digest our food, it sinks into the unconscious. Only disorders such as cramps, heaviness, or pain make us pay attention to the digestive organs. These are the signal that there is something we urgently have to change about the way we see our body.

In the last ten years, many studies have appeared that link the billions of microbes on our body, health, and well-being. The direct or indirect implication of microbes in an impressive number of diseases in the modern world supports the fact that we are at the peak of a paradigm shift concerning conventional notions of health and disease.

What makes the role of the intestinal microbiota so fascinating and so far-reaching is the fact that this mass of microorganisms binds precisely to the interface that separates our physical reactions and sensations. The bacteria in our intestines play an important role in terms of mood, the tendency to socialize, and even the food choices of each one of us.

We can already guess that, if we want to reach a certain level of well-being, we must be able to count on their collaboration. Since biblical times great importance has been given to the action of fermented foods and the bacteria they contain. And the remarkable age of Abraham was reduced to the regular consumption of products based on lactic acid.

Recalling the millenary food tradition of all the people of the earth and taking advantage of ancient Eastern wisdom, beneficial microbes such as Lactobacilli and Bifidobacterium, which are seen in fermented foods can improve the differentiation of our intestinal microbial ecosystem.

In this thesis we will see how intestinal bacteria affect our behavior and our psychophysical well-being, how they influence our thoughts, our emotions, our relationship with others, even our vision of the world, but also how these bacteria, and therefore our global health depends strictly on the type of diet and lifestyle we choose to adopt.

Once we have embarked on this path of awareness that the host-microbe relationship is an integral part of the wider biosphere, we can begin to think about health as part of a socio-ecological system and provide a ramp to connect the points.

Chapter 1

INTESTINAL MICROCOSM

OUR (SECOND) BRAIN THAT WORKS BY BACTERIA

By our digestive versatility, we have managed to ensure sustenance in the most varied conditions of our climate and environment. Millions of years of evolution have refined the ability of the intestine to perceive, recognize and codify all that we eat and drink in patterns of hormonal and nervous impulses that are sent to the regulatory centers of the brain.

If the intestine was once considered a small digestive organ, today we know that it can actively intervene even in the sphere of emotions. It does not decide if we only digest food well or badly, and if they are transformed into fat pads on our sides, but it also illuminates our "internal situation."

Popular wisdom has known for a long time: we are talking about "decisions taken with the stomach," stress and annoyances often "close our stomachs" or "don't go down." When we are afraid, "we can do it," while happiness manifests itself with "butterflies in the stomach." And sometimes some things make us "throw up."

There is no other organ that reacts so quickly to our emotions as the intestine. The center of the body is very closely connected to the world of feelings, which is why we speak of an "enteric brain." But how can a portion of the mucosa, grazed by more or less interesting stools, be able to think?

DECIDING HOW WE ARE THREE LARGE "UNITS" IN THE INTESTINE CONTROL ROOM:

• The innumerable nerve cells present in the intestine, which are in a very close relationship with the brain;

• The chemical messengers, which are mostly produced in the gastrointestinal tract, but can fully perform their activities also in the brain;

• The billions of intestinal bacteria that stir our emotions with zeal and influences our mood, appetite, and well-being in various ways.

The nervous system is a means of communication used by the intestinal bacteria. The vagus nerve, the longest of the twelve cranial nerves, is the main channel of communication between the neurons of the intestinal nervous system and those of the central nervous system. This nerve extends to the base of the brain up to the abdomen. The bacteria intervenes by secreting some neurotransmitters similar to those produced by the brain. Neurotransmitters, chemical messengers, represent, in a certain sense, the words with which belly and brain dialogue with each other.

They stimulate the 12 neurons of the intestine, or enteric neurons, which in turn communicate with the brain neurons via the vagus nerve. The interesting thing is that almost ninety percent of the nerve fibers goes only in one direction, which is to the brain, and only ten percent of the information runs from the head to the intestine.

It means that the belly exploits this last highway of data to tell the head what is happening down there. Through blood or nerve impulses, they reach the gray matter, but they do not activate in all areas of the brain. The neurotransmitters that come from the intestine are well placed in the areas responsible for emotions, learning, and motivation. The limbic system, with the hippocampus and amygdala, is among their favorite destinations.

The intestine acts autonomously, that is, it is independent, it manages its work, and is not subjected to the orders of the brain. That digestion is an unconscious process, of course, is a great fortune. If our brain were to direct every single stimulus of the intestine consciously, we could not devote ourselves to any other activity, because we would always be busy digesting.

We are not aware of the ongoing communicative exchanges between the intestine and the brain, nor are we aware of the chemical messengers that the first sends to the second. They can change our view of the reality in which we live.

They can make us happy or fearful, lead to depression or even physical ailments. Perhaps even diseases like autism, Parkinson's disease, and hyperactivity are closely linked to what goes on in our bowels. Nature has programmed humans to distinguish different emotions and react accordingly easily.

They are so obvious because the brain sends a clear pattern of signals to the many small muscles of the face, which means that every emotion has a facial correspondence, and someone nearby can identify it. Each of us is an open book. However, we are blind to the intestinal manifestations of these emotions.

When we are furious because of the traffic, our brain, just like it does with the facial muscles, transmits a series of signals to the digestive system, which also has an intense reaction. The intestinal mucosa is dotted with endocrine cells, specialized units containing up to twenty different types of hormones that can be released into the bloodstream if necessary.

If it were possible to bring them all together in one mass, its dimensions would be greater than those of all the other endocrine organs, gonads, thyroid, pituitary, and adrenal glands, put together.

If the only task of the intestine is to govern digestion, why would such a quantity of specialized cells count? Our intestine has a crucial function as a large sensory organ covering the greater part of our body. Its surface is equal to that of a basketball field, and in it, there are thousands of small sensors that encode the vast number of information present in food in the form of signaling molecules, from sweet to bitter, from hot to cold and from spicy to tasteless.

Many of the signals of the intestine to the brain does not only generate sensations like those of satiety and well-being after a good meal, nausea or discomfort but also provoke responses of the brain to the intestine, giving rise to distinct somatic reactions. And the brain does not forget these sensations.

They are stored in large brain databases that can be accessed when decisions are made. What we feel in the intestine ends up influencing not only our preferences in terms of food and drink but also about the people we choose to spend time with and how we evaluate crucial information as workers, jury members or leaders.

According to MTC (Medicine traditional Chinese) in Chinese philosophy, the concept of yin and yang describes opposing or contrary forces that can be considered complementary and interconnected, and that give rise to a unified whole by interacting with each other. By applying this idea to the intestine - brain axis, we can consider somatic and yang reactions as somatic reactions.

As yin and yang are the two complementary principles of the same entity, so the sensations and reactions are different aspects of the same bidirectional brain-intestine system that plays such an essential role in our well-being, in our emotions and in our ability to make intuitive decisions.

For traditional Chinese medicine (TCM) in the theory of five movements, the heart and small intestine belong to the Fire Lodge. The discernment of thoughts also takes place in the heart. Every thought, before being implemented, it will be analyzed by the heart that discerns it, hence, separating what is good from what is bad.

On the psychic level, what is carried out on the physical plane by the small intestine where the substances considered good (absorbed) are separated from those considered not good (eliminated).

The large intestine belongs to the metal loggia and is associated with the lung. In TCM, the symbolic and energetic meaning is considered beyond the organic structure of the lung and large intestine. Breathing is a fundamental function for life and the organic functions of the whole organism. With the breath, the energy, the emotions, and the waste substances are expelled into us as well as the air with its chemical components, useless and harmful to our body and negative emotions, many times deep breaths together with positive visualizations can help to overcome moments of anxiety and fear.

The functions of the large intestine are similar and not by chance, they are in the same lodge: it absorbs the beneficial substances and expels the body's waste, allowing the body to grow and purify itself. When for various situations the intestine holds back instead of eliminating there are many disorders such as swelling, constipation, colds, acne, headache; also the emotional closure and therefore the difficulty in letting go of the emotions is connected to a malfunction of the intestine.

INTESTINAL MICROBIOTE, A SENSORY ORGANIC COMPOUND

Bacteria and microorganisms are omnipresent: they live on the skin, in the nose, and the intestine. Our gastrointestinal system, particularly the large intestine, is home to far more diverse populations. From the scientific point of view, doctors describe the complexity of microorganisms that live in humans with the term microbiota.

In recent times, medicine has shown much interest in life within the intestine; some have called it a "forgotten organ." A person's alimentary canal is the most densely populated ecosystem on Earth. About one hundred trillion microbes (bacteria, viruses, fungi) roam on the surface of the substantially oxygen-free intestine. It is a huge number, unimaginable, written in numbers, it corresponds to 100,000,000,000,000 and is a thousand times greater than the number of stars that make up our galaxy.

If we put together all our intestinal microbes giving them the shape of an organ, this would weigh from 0.9 to 2.7 kg, compared to the brain weighing 1.2 kg. First, there was the talk of bacterial "flora" in the intestine. But this concept does not do justice to reality. The word flora is originated from the Latin, and it indicates the growth of plants on a portion of land, therefore something static.

Plants always remain in the same place. The concept of "bacterial flora" dates back to the period in which it was imagined that bacteria grew on the mucosa like grass on the earth and that the inside of the body was not touched. For this reason, we also talked about "bacterial carpet." Today we know that we are a dynamic whole and bacteria penetrate inside us, penetrating us. They do not generate only in portions of the border. Everywhere, on and in our bodies, the surfaces, the passages between the inside and the outside are covered with biofilms of bacteria which in turn are formed by microbes that remain, comes and goes in a dynamic process. In the wake of the pioneering of the Human Genome Project, which has identified every human gene, scientists are now able to sequence large amounts of DNA very quickly and cheaply.

Now it is even possible to identify dead microbes expelled from the body in defecation because their DNA remains intact. We felt that our microbes were not important, but science is beginning to reveal a different story to us. A story in which human life is intertwined with that of our hitchhikers, in which microbes manage the body, and it is not possible for the human body to be healthy without them.

How many genes are needed to form a human being? From the hypotheses of the group of the most prepared people on the planet surely a higher number, compared to the number of genes of the mice, which as we knew had 23,000.

With its timid 21,000 genes, the human genome is not much larger than that of a worm. It is half that of the rice plant, and even the simple water flea with 31,000 genes outclasses it. Certainly, a complex and sophisticated body like the human body needs more proteins, and therefore more genes, than that of a worm.

But these 21,000 genes are not the only genes that govern our body. We do not live alone. Each of us is a superorganism. Our cells, although much larger in weight and volume, are outnumbered in numbers, in the proportion of ten to one, by the cells of the microbes that live in and above us. Altogether, the microbes that live on the human body contain 4.4 million genes: here is the microbiome, the collective genome of the microbiota.

The Human Microbiome Project (HMP), a consortium of 200 researchers from 80 US research institutions in 5 years, analyzed the genome of microbes living on the human body, the microbiome, to identify which species are present.

From this variety of microorganisms, about 70% is located in the gastrointestinal tract with a concentration that increases exponentially in the fecal-oral direction. All this population can be divided into two large groups:

1. The autochthonous bacteria that start to colonize the digestive tract from birth and, after weaning, they turn into permanent, stable colonies. The quality and quantity of some particular strains can provide such constant "imprinting" that it can be used for individual identification with a precision higher than that of fingerprints!

2. The allochthones bacteria is found in our intestine only in a short form without forming stable colonies, and they are introduced with food when their number increases they cause imbalances that from simple dysbiosis can reach even more serious diseases. As we proceed inside the gastrointestinal system, the environmental conditions change, and this determines the variety of microbial species that settle at different levels. The bacteria colonize the segments of the intestinal tube where they find the most suitable conditions for their development: however, anatomy and physiology are essential in determining the quantity and quality of microorganisms. In general, traits, where the contractile movement of the intestine (peristalsis) is more contained, are welcome.

Among the factors that regulate the balance of the bacterial population is the pH, which is the acidity or basicity of the environment, oxygen, nutrients, and the presence of competitors. All the bacteria that live in the gastrointestinal tract are also found in the faeces whose composition reproduces the balance that has been established in recent stretches. In inflammatory bowel diseases, and not only, instead of a functioning microbiome, there is also a disorder in the intestinal microbes, and the result is an excess or defect of metabolic products, genetic activations, and enzymes.

This condition is called "dysbiosis." The term originated from the Greek words dys for "wrong," "disturbed" and bios for "life" and the ending "-osi" for "condition," "state." A simple way to identify a dysbiosis is the control of the stool surfacing in the toilet (correct eubiosis) compared to a sinking (dysbiosis in progress).

THE INTESTINAL MICROBIOTE IN FIGURES
• 100,000 billion bacteria •

The number of intestinal bacteria is equal to 10 times the cells present in our body • about 1000 different bacterial species (each has 160 to 200) • A real organ that weighs as much as the liver or the brain (from 1 to 2 Kg)

Chapter 2

WHERE DO OUR INTESTINAL BACTERIA COME FROM?

Human beings, since the beginning of their evolution, have lived in constant association with bacteria: we can, therefore, consider them as our "oldest friends," a true "presence," for many years neglected by scientific research and undervalued in the therapeutic protocols. To fully understand the extraordinary importance of the role of microbes in our body, it is worth remembering where they come from and how they connected with us.

For about 3 billion years ago, bacteria were the only living beings on the planet. They occupied every strip of land, air, and water, creating the conditions for the development of multicellular life with chemical reactions. Gradually, by trial and error through the vastness of time, they invented the complex and solid feedback systems, including the very effective "language" that has so far supported all life on earth. Our colony begins with Noah's ark of species, given to us by our mother at birth. Our mother's first microbes, of course, came from our grandmother and so on till infinity. In the indefinite universe of 8000 generations ago, microbial gift was passed down from mother to son in our pre-Homo Sapiens ancestors.

In the context of our evolutionary history, this transfer goes back beyond humanity, beyond primates, even beyond mammals, to reach the dawn of the animal kingdom. One of the favorite tricks of biology teachers is to ask students to spread their arms and trace the biography of the planet in the extension between the two hands. On the tip of the middle finger of the right is the formation of the earth, 4.6 billion years ago. The tip of the left hand represents the current world. The earth cools down more or less at the right elbow, and life begins in the form of bacteria. From these simple beginnings, it is almost necessary to reach the left wrist, 3 billion years later, for simpler animals to evolve.

Mammals, in all their hairy and thoughtful glory, have reached more or less the left index, and humans like us have come forward just a hair from the nail of that finger. It has already been said: a stroke of a file and every trace of our existence would vanish.

Animals, therefore, have never known life without bacteria. Their existence is so intertwined that inside (almost) every cell of every animal, ghost cells of the simplest bacteria have been inserted. Enveloped by a larger cell, these bacteria earn hospitality worthily, because each specializes in producing energy from food molecules. They are our mitochondria, the power stations of cells, which convert food into energy thanks to cellular respiration. Fundamental to multicellular life, now as in the early days of the animal kingdom, these former bacteria have become so entrenched that we no longer consider them even microbes. Mitochondria represent an evolutionary signature of the first alliances between two organisms.

Just as in the sixteenth century, the Copernican revolution fundamentally changed our knowledge of the position of the earth in the solar system, and the revolutionary theory formulated by Darwin in the nineteenth century forever changed our position in the animal kingdom. The science of the human microbiome is there forcing once more to reconsider the place we occupy on the planet.

According to this new science, we are superorganisms, composed of strictly interconnected human and microbial elements, inseparable and dependent on each other for survival. And the most interesting fact is that the microbial contribution to this superorganism is enormously greater than ours.

Since the microbial component, through a common biological communication system, is so intimately connected with all the other microbiomes present in the soil, in the air and in the sea, and with the microbes that live in symbiosis with almost all other living creatures, we are intrinsically and inextricably connected with the terrestrial network of life. The new concept of human microbial superorganism has profound implications for our understanding of the role we play on the planet, and of many aspects of health and disease.

In the course of life, we host so many microbes that in 20 realities, we are not individuals but colonies. Our skin is teeming with it. On the fingers, there is a greater number of the population of Great Britain.

Variable and dynamic like our rotating planet, the human body has a chemical climate that increases and decreases depending on the hormonal tides, and of complex passages that change with the passing of the years. For microbes, this is Eden. Our perception of the microorganisms residing in our body is slowly evolving.

Until recently, we talked about bacteria only because of their pathogenic appearance, and how harmful or friendly they can be. In fact, in the not too distant past, bacterial infections such as measles, hepatitis, or tuberculosis were one of the main causes of deaths globally. Starting from Pasteur's studies, the aspiration to a "sterile" world in which man would have won his battle against any microbes, which would have ended with their extermination, has spread.

Today there is a radical change of perspective. We realized that the vast majority of bacteria play a beneficial role for humans. They are part of us, and genetically speaking, 99% are our friends. We, as superorganisms, live in symbiosis with them. We need each other to live.

A FIRST FINGER OF OUR INTESTINAL MICROBIOTA

There is a direct link between the state of the intestinal microbiota and our mind from birth. According to some neuroscientists, this connection would also be because the bacteria present in the intestine, producing a lot of DNA, synthesize molecules. For a complex mechanism of immune, hormonal, and neural mediation, they modulate brain development both in fetal life and throughout life.

Colonization occurs at the time of birth, and the first pattern of the bacteria depends on the type of birth, feeding, and environmental conditions. Food plays an essential role in the health of the intestine, the brain, and in the interaction between these two vital organs, and this close relationship also begins at the moment of birth.

While it is true that as adults we all want optimal health, let's not forget that some of the most important influences of food on the microbiome start long before we can make our decisions about what to eat and which probiotics to choose. These early food-related influences on the intestinal microbiome lay the foundation for our adult intestinal microbial diversity and our resistance to disease, and errors in the process of this original programming can increase the potential risks to our health.

A study by the microbiologist Ruth Ley and her team at Cornell University, highlighted the remarkable influence of the early stages of nourishment on the intestinal microbiota of a healthy child. The study was carried out sixty times, from the child's birth to about two and a half years. For the first four and a half months, the baby was exclusively breastfed. In the beginning, they discovered that his microbiota was rich in microbial species that facilitated the digestion of milk carbohydrates, primarily Bifidobacterium and some Lactobacilli. However, before the subject began to consume powdered milk or any solid food, intestinal microbes such as the prevotella appeared; (prevotella is capable of metabolizing complex carbohydrates from vegetables). It implies that the baby's gut microbiota was ready for solid food even before it started to consume them. The mother continued to breastfeed her until she was nine months old, and the parents gradually introduced baby food such as rice and peas, when the baby switched to solid foods, the microbiota turned back into microbes capable of fermenting vegetable carbohydrates.

In the first two months of the child's life, a relatively low number of species lived in his gut and events such as a fever, the introduction of peas in the diet or an antibiotic-based treatment for otitis caused some major fluctuations in the microbial communities. However, the diversity recovered within a month, and by the age of two and a half the microbiome had now stabilized and resembled that of an adult.

Based on this and other studies, it is now clear that a human's first two and a half to three years shape the intestinal microbiome throughout life. It is as if the child's body composed a symphony orchestra, in which each species of intestinal bacteria plays a single instrument. At first, the players try. Some are hired, others are not, but many places remain empty. At the age of two and a half, however, the orchestra is complete, and most of the players retain their lifetime employment. Depending on the circumstances and food reserves, the orchestra can play an entire repertoire of different motifs.

The mechanisms by which intestinal microbiota can be influenced from the beginning of life are numerous, and they include feeding the mother during pregnancy and lactation, exposure to environmental microbes and brain-intestinal signals induced by the stress that attracts the intestinal microbiome of both the mother and the newborn. The geographical differences in the composition of the microbiota could also be due to the significant differences in the environmental conditions of individuals living in harmony with their environment in remote parts of the world. Compared to residents in the metropolitan areas that are far from direct exposure to the natural environment, and who consume their food at the restaurant or buys it in supermarkets.

People living in industrialized societies have a "restrictive" composition of intestinal microbiota, which is not as efficient in fermenting complex carbohydrates derived from plants into short chain fatty acids, even if we consume many plant-derived foods. It may be due to the absence of some microbial species such as the bacterium Ruminococcus bromii, whose activities are essential to initiate the breakdown of these difficult-to-break substrates.

Within the intestinal microbiota ecosystem, many of the same metabolites can be produced by different members of the microbial community, and are consumed or transformed by others. Different species of intestinal microbes possess more specialized abilities and appear to play a key role in degrading the starch particles that escape digestion in the small intestine.

All this means that when we are born in Western civilization, we also acquire their microbiome. Even if today I decided to become vegan, my intestinal microbiota will remain that typical of an omnivore, and even if we adhered to a Paleolithic diet for the rest of our lives, our microbiota would never turn into a hunter-gatherer.

However, the pattern of microbial metabolites we produce depends on the diet we follow. Even if a friend of mine and I follow a similar diet, we will have different species of microbes in the intestine. Each of us shares only a small amount of microbial species and strains with other humans. Although two grasslands appear to be similar in photography, compared to two forests, they may differ greatly due to the hundreds of species of plants and animals that live in them and that create these environments with a similar appearance.

Chapter 3

THE LANGUAGE OF MICROBES: AN ESSENTIAL COMPONENT OF DIALOGUE BETWEEN INTESTINE AND BRAIN

Roth and LeRoith summarized their findings in an article published in the New England Journal of Medicine, stating that the signaling molecules used by the endocrine system and the brain to communicate probably originated from microbes. As we understand it now, this invisible mass of life can continuously communicate with the brain using a variety of signals, including hormones, neurotransmitters, and a myriad of small compounds called metabolites.

The latter is the result of the peculiar eating habits of microbes, which generate them when they feed on the indigestible residues of what we consume, of bile acids secreted by the liver in the intestine or of the layer of mucus that covers the intestine. In the conversation between the brain and intestine, the intestinal microbiota engages in a structured and continuous dialogue using a sophisticated biochemical code, the "language of microbes." Why do gut microbes and the brain need such a sophisticated communication system? How does the language of microbes develop? I have searched far back in time to the primordial seas of the earth rich in microorganisms.

The symbiosis between small sea creatures and their resident microbes brought many advantages to both. Animals acquired the ability to digest certain foods, obtain vitamins that they could not synthesize on their own, and avoid or expel toxins and other environmental hazards. The microbes of their digestive system had a controlled and comfortable environment in which to thrive and free movement from one point to another. That set of microorganisms can be considered the first version of the intestinal microbiota. The symbiotic relationship between the intestinal microbes and their hosts proved to be so beneficial for both partners that it was maintained in virtually every multicellular animal that lives on earth today.

The major digestive activities have been continued for hundreds of millions of years, this attests to the extraordinary evolutionary intelligence that has been programmed in our intestine and the enteric system (SNE) and makes it even more logical why there is such an intricate link between our microbes, the intestine, and the brain.

The SNE includes more neurons than the spinal cord, and from its development, we can see that it has to do with our feelings: it is derived from cells that move along the vagus nerve in the intestine in the embryonic development and then differentiate into nerve cells. Their origin is the limbic system which, from the history of evolution, is an ancient part of the cerebral cortex in which feelings and emotions are processed. The SNE grew up moving from head to belly. No wonder the two parts are related to each other. Hundreds of millions of years have passed since a handful of microbes established the first contact with the primitive gut of a simple marine animal. But the long evolutionary journey that we have undertaken since then has helped to explain why today our intestine, with its enteric nervous system and its microbiome, continues to exert such a significant influence on our emotions and our general well-being.

The amount of information that can travel with this system depends largely on the thickness and integrity of the thin layer of mucus that lines the surface of the intestine, the permeability of the intestinal wall and the blood-brain barrier.

Under normal conditions, these natural barriers are relatively impermeable, and the flow of data from intestinal microbes to the brain is limited. However, stress, inflammation, a high-fat diet, and certain food additives can make them more permeable.

What makes the role of the intestinal microbiota so fascinating and so far-reaching is the fact that this mass of microorganisms binds precisely to the interface that separates our reactions and somatic sensations. The bacteria in our intestines play an important role in terms of mood, the tendency to socialize, and even the food choices of each of us. We can already guess that, if we want to reach a certain level of well-being, we must be able to count on their collaboration. How do these bacteria always communicate with our body and influence it so profoundly? What means do they use to communicate and act?

The brain receives the information generated by the trillions of microbes that live there, an aspect of brain-intestinal communication that has only been focused in recent years. Scientists call the continuous reports on the state of the body "interoceptive" information that the brain uses to maintain the balance and regular functioning of the body systems. Even if this information comes from every cell, the messages sent to the brain from the intestine and its neural mechanisms are unique in terms of numbers, variety, and complexity.

To begin with, let us consider that the neural network of our intestines is distributed over its entire surface, which is two hundred times larger than that of the skin. If we consider the dense distribution of receptors and the vast area they occupy on the lining of the intestine wall, it is clear that the latter transmits a huge mass of data to the brain at any time, both from the complicated processes related to digestion and from input of 100 trillion microbes that chatter in our intestinal tract.

When it comes to collecting, storing, analyzing, and responding to large amounts of information, the Cerebro-intestinal axis is a true supercomputer, and it is very different from the slow steam machine to which it was once compared. This awareness is part of our new, modern knowledge of intestinal function, which implies that, the transition from concern for macro and micronutrient details, metabolism and calories to the understanding that our gut, with its nervous system and its microbes, is actually an extraordinary computer that extensively exceeds the brain in terms of the number of cells involved, and equals some of its capabilities.

Through the foods we consume, this system intimately connects us to the world around us, gathering information on how our food is grown, what we put in the soil to get it and which chemicals were added before we bought it at the supermarket to preserve it.

Intestinal microbes play a significant role in this connection between what we eat and how we feel. Beyond the undeniable fact that the two nervous and enteric systems are in communication with each other, a third important actor also enters the intestinal microbiota. At this point, it is legitimate to speak of a microbiota-intestine-brain axis.

WHAT DO THE BACTERIA DO FOR US?

The intestinal bacteria produce substances that act on the brain through the intestinal mucosa and cover different ways: blood, immune, and nervous. They carry out an enormous metabolic job and constitute a precious ecosystem that, if intact, is very important for health and well-being.

"The microbiota can be seen as a metabolic" organ "tuned to our physiology." (Backhed, 2004) They play a vital role in the digestion, assimilation, and elimination of food. Without bacteria it would be impossible to digest certain types of fiber properly. They feed and digest them for us, and in doing so, they also produce some nutrients we need. Depending on the diet, the bacteria release a particular amount of active metabolic substances. The vitamins belong to these. Certain Bifidus and Escherichia Coli strains produce, as it was discovered in 1983, vitamins of the B group: B1, B2, B3 and their nicotinamide derivatives, B5, B6, B12, folic acid, biotin and vitamin K necessary for blood coagulation.

For their metabolism, for example, nerve cells need vitamin B12 and folic acid, both of which are supplied by food through the action of intestinal bacteria. Even a minimal deficiency of these trace elements can cause an insufficient supply to the nerves which have repercussions in the form of nervous weakness in the belly-brain-belly agreement. For example, they collaborate in the synthesis of vitamin D, which is essential for proper bone mineralization and the adequate functioning of the immune system.

The intestinal bacteria also perform a detoxifying function, neutralizing, for example, some substances that are harmful to our body, such as ammonia. The unhealthy microbiota developed, increases the levels of pro-inflammatory cytokines, such as IL-6 and IL-8 and lipopolysaccharide (LPS), which cause intestinal inflammation and permeability of the walls.

Furthermore, these inflammatory molecules contribute to the metabolic dysfunction with the altered metabolism of bile acid, the production of short-chain fatty acids, the secretion of the intestinal hormone, and the circulation of branched-chain amino acids. The most important role bacteria play in the reabsorption of bile acids. Bile is composed of bile salts, the bilirubin dye, cholesterol, and phospholipids. These are important for bile stabilization. If the bile is salty, bilirubin or cholesterol crystallize, gallstones form, based on their relationship with phospholipids. Bile is formed in liver cells and the gall bladder and from there, depending on food intake, released into the small intestine. Bile also contains several enzymes and substances that the liver has filtered to purify the body.

If the intestine is not healthy, it can leave the liver with a more significant number of toxic substances through the bile to detoxify, then brought back into the intestine, through which they should be eliminated. If the microbiome is in good shape here, the intestinal bacteria carry out the steps necessary for detoxification; otherwise, they may be reabsorbed and returned to the liver.

Great attention was paid to the possible role of short chain fatty acids (SCFA acronym for Short Chain Fatty Acids) such as butyrate, propionate, and acetate since SCFA are the main product of the digestive action of intestinal microbiota. It has been reported that SCFAs affect host metabolism through various parallel pathways associated with protein-coupled receptors, and these receptors are active in neuroendocrine cells in the intestine and can, therefore, influence brain signaling. Recent studies has shown differences in the ratio of the three essential fatty acids between them. While in healthy subjects all fatty acids (acetic acid, propionic acid, butyric acid) should be present in a relationship of about 60: 25: 10%, in patients with Crohn's disease they were in a ratio of 70: 15: 8%.

Based on the type and quantity of food, chewing, and time spent on meals, these secretions are in smaller or larger quantities. Furthermore, the more consciously a meal is taken, the more adequate the amount of juices secreted with the food taken will be. The gut's bacteria part in the reabsorption of these glandular secretions is so important for the body, in which there are also complex bonds such as those of hormones.

It has been shown that butyric acid and propionic acid inhibit the growth of cancer cells. Increasing their quantity through bacteria in the intestine could be part of successful cancer therapy. In a healthy microbiome, the various bioactive substances, which are formed through the bacteria of the intestine, contributes to the body's nutrition, in a gut with incorrect colonization; instead, they carry cellular damage.

The more a disturbance persists in the intestinal mucosa, in the form of a reduction in the number of microbes, a modified composition, a lack of mucosa, inflammation, immune reactions and the higher the probability that the cells of the intestinal epithelium do what they want.

In most cases, this all starts in the lower part of the large intestine, in the rectum. Mecnikov, director of the Pasteur Institute in Paris (1845-1916) discussed the proposal to "simply eliminate the large intestine with an operation to avoid the harmful effects of intestinal microbes living in this useless organ." Since on the other hand, Mecnikov had observed that the bacterial flora in newborns changed after drinking breast milk for the first time and that this would be different from that of babies fed with cow's milk.

Mecnikov concluded that nutrition influences the intestinal microbes. This led him to the idea of altering our flora to replace harmful microbes with 29 other profits through a varied diet. In search of similar foods, he came across fermented dairy products. The path of the reflections that Mecnikov had made at the time, namely to avoid operations using a modified diet favorable to microbes for a better intestinal bacterial colonization, can still help to move away from the need for an operation, to cure polyps and tumors intestinal via a change in the intestinal microbiome.

For nerve cells to at least be able to transmit impulses to other cells, communication, a compatible instrument is necessary for everyone. These are nerve messengers, neurotransmitters. Small molecules that are transported by a nerve cell in the space of the next one. Serotonin is one of the most vital neurotransmitters, and it is found mainly in the intestine. Its effects on the body affect all central, and vital areas: like the heart and circulation of blood coagulation, or regulation of eye pressure. It transmits mucosal stimuli to the tissues in the gastrointestinal tract, and as a result of this, the movements of the organs are coordinated. Also, it occurs directly or indirectly, in almost all the functions of the central nervous system and of the enteric ones: the serotonin rule perception, sensitivity and temperature, tiredness and pain, stimulus development, hormonal production, and sexual behavior.

If there is enough serotonin in the body, the human being is balanced, if the serotonin is lacking, moods appear as prostration and killing, up to depression, dissatisfaction, irritability, fear, and aggressive behavior. It also performs protective functions and increases the barrier effect: increased production of mucin and zoludin is a component of the tight junctions (the tight junctions that allow the intestinal epithelium to act as a protective barrier towards the inside of the body).

Finally, the intestinal microbiota is essential for our immune system. About 70-80% of the body's immune cells are located in the intestine. The microbiota stimulates the maturation of the immune system and has a "barrier effect" against potential aggressors. The "good" bacteria (saprophytes or commensals) attach themselves to the intestinal wall and occupy the space, thus preventing the establishment of harmful bacteria.

Bacteria make the nerves grow or prevent its growth, and they make the connections grow or prevent them, inhibit, favor, or regulate. Bacteria determine brain activity, the values of blood and tissues of neurotransmitters, hormones, and hematocytes, as well as development and inflammation and vegetative reactions, depend on them. Intestinal bacteria is the part that accompanies us throughout our lives, and the brain development of our ability to feel, to behave and even to think, without them, we will not be a whole human being.

Some microorganisms can produce a neurotransmitter, gamma-aminobutyric acid. This substance, abbreviated as GABA, is one of the most abundant signaling molecules in the nervous system, which keeps the emotional part of our brain, the limbic system, under control. But it would be possible to use this knowledge to treat anxiety disorders with GABA-producing microbes in the form of probiotics.

We know that some strains of two of the most studied families of beneficial intestinal bacteria, Lactobacilli, and Bifidobacterium, have the potential to produce synthetic GABA. Since different bacterial strains of these two families are active ingredients in the most common probiotics, and both groups tend to abound in fermented food products.

Could it be possible that further addition of these microbes to our diet makes us feel more relaxed? Could a regime as simple as fermented foods help apprehensive individuals to reduce their anxiety levels?

Chapter 4

THE CONSEQUENCES OF AN UNBALANCED INTESTINAL MICROBIOTE ON OUR WELL-BEING

In the case of dysbiosis caused by excessive proliferation of harmful bacteria or poor differentiation of bacterial strains, the microbiota will produce harmful effects on the rest of the body and then to the brain. The "bad" bacteria will produce toxic substances, called "neurotoxins," for the nervous system.

These neurotoxins will eventually alter mental functions, generating stress, anxiety, and even psychiatric or neurodegenerative diseases. An imbalance in the intestinal microbiota will have the effect of depleting or over-stimulating the immune system. The harmful bacteria that prevail over those beneficial alters of the intestinal wall can make it porous, allowing the passage of macromolecules and foreign toxins into the blood.

These intruders cause the immediate reaction of intestinal immune cells, which will alert the entire immune system, releasing inflammatory molecules and stress hormones. In this way, the harmful intestinal bacteria can start a state of chronic inflammation, with negative effects on the brain and our mental health.

Dr. Hiromi Shinya, the author of the book "Microbes and Immunity," maintains that 30% of the intestinal microbiota consists of beneficial bacteria's which act in our favor. 20% of pathogenic bacteria and the remaining 50% of neutral bacteria, to determine their behavior, more or less beneficial for human cells, will be the soil on which they will develop, determined mainly by what we eat and the lifestyle we adopt.

The instability of the intestinal ecosystem depends on many factors:

1. Physiological factors, such as an unsuitable diet

2. Pathological factors, such as acute and chronic intestinal diseases, systemic pathologies, hormonal alterations, stress, immunological diseases, liver diseases.

3. The iatrogenic factors, such as synthetic surgical interventions, antibiotics, analgesics and antiphlogistic, chemical additives (to keep in mind that in the case of antibiotics and other drugs. Their intake can also occur through organic products, for example, meat, fish, or eggs, derived from animals that have been treated with these substances).

When the intestinal ecosystem alters, the mucosa becomes the site of inflammation, and digestion is insufficient, intestinal hygiene becomes precarious, the defective immune system and hormone production is impaired. The most common manifestations concern different systems, from the gastrointestinal to the respiratory system, from the skin to the osteoarticular because the mechanism of inflammation can develop in any part of the body.

However the most frequent symptoms are: meteorism, abdominal swellings, irregular alvo, acne, breathlessness, canker sores, anxiety, asthma, headache, cellulite, colic, diarrhea, insomnia, eczema, headaches, irritable bowel, hives, eczema, itching, drowsiness, overweight, water retention, constipation, flatulence, belching, aerophagia, and feeling of nausea, dermatitis, and urticaria.

Unsuitable foods can generate digestion at altered pH (vaccines, infections, antibiotics, and generally all drugs, too much alcohol, coffee, etc.) irritate the internal lining of the epithelial mucosa of the intestine. Hence, making it inflamed and overexcited, damaging it and making it porous, opening small breaches in the walls that allow the passage of bacteria, fungi and toxic substances (macromolecules) in the blood, which is recognized by the body as possible antigenic agents, causing abnormal reactions of the immune system.

The intestinal dysbiotic-fermentative alterations that occur mainly at the level of the colon due to poor diet produce toxins which, through the vascular system, are fixed in the Extra Cellular Matrix (ECM). The colloidal toxins which are molecules that are too large to pass through the membranes; their task is to push liquids into the intravascular space, and the crystalloids which are solutions containing electrolytes that move freely between the intravascular compartments and between the interstitial spaces; they have the same concentration of electrolytes of extracellular liquids for which they do not alter the plasma. When they are absorbed, they cause metabolic alterations due to their acidifying action and cellular oxidation with consequent slowing of metabolic exchanges and interstitial water retention.

How can you personally determine the conditions your microbiome is located? The variables are many like the several types of bacteria, what you eat, the climate, and your lifestyle — paradoxically returning to do what the same Hippocratic medicine did, and which is also practiced in the Chinese medicine, specifically to observe the person, and what the body shows, returning to learn how to decode the language, treating signs and symptoms as a communication code and not as a mere annoyances to be suppressed.

A healthy microbiome is not just felt. Painful swellings, cramps, intestinal gas or signs of intolerance are already suggestive of the disorder. Stool observation is essential as is control of the oral mucosa. The consistency of the stool can provide indications on the size of the microbiome disorder. The form of the faeces that are released is formally the creative expression of the intestine and therefore of the whole inner life.

In 1997 the doctors of the Bristol University Clinic in England divided the faeces into the following scale of seven types: •

Type 1: single hard lumps similar to hazelnuts (difficult to evacuate);

Type 2: salami-shaped and knotty;

Type 3: salami-shaped with surface cracks;

Type 4: snail-shaped without shell, smooth and soft;

Type 5: soft piles with smooth edges (easy to evacuate);

Type 6: loose pieces with irregular, pasty contours;

Type 7: aqueous without stable structures.

This scale, known as the "Bristol Stool Chart," is a good reference point for identifying microbiome trends. Types 3 and 4 are considered to be normal stools, types 1 and 2 indicate constipation and types 5, 6, and 7 indicate dysentery. When these last appear permanently, as well as when there is a continuous change in the consistency of the stools, it can be an indication of a disorder of the microbiome.

Digestive disorders can be recognized in the faeces through the presence of food remains, mucous patina, sticky, greasy or shiny surfaces, but even through a different color or smell of putrid. Healthy stools are normally odorless. In order not to cause a new shock to the microbiome, it is better to gradually replace the previous diet with the new one, so that the right intestinal bacteria can multiply in harmony.

Chapter 5
CAUSES OF DYSBIOSIS INTESTINAL IATROGENE

- Antibiotic therapy
- Immunodepression
- Psych pharmaceuticals
- Oral contraceptives
- Ionizing radiations

FOOD

- Unilateral unbalanced diet
- Additives, antibiotics, growth stimulators
- Food preservatives and dyes
- Denatured foods

BOWEL

- Malabsorption
- Inflammation
- PH alteration
- Pancreatitis

• Intestinal infections

PSYCHIC

• Stress &Anxiety

• Concern

SYMBIOTICS FOR THE RESTORATION OF THE INTESTINAL EQUILIBRIUM

For some years now, scientific research has paid attention to the combination of probiotics and prebiotics, the so-called symbiotic, by their multiple possibilities of use. Probiotics are microorganisms that exert a positive effect on the balance of the microbiota, and prebiotics are substances that supply energy to bacteria.

Combining, these microorganisms promote the specific multiplication of bacteria essential for the life of the intestine and stimulate their activity and the possibility of survival. In this case, symbiotics can help restore the balance of our intestines.

• PROBIOTICS; According to the definition of the World Health Organization, probiotics are live micro-organisms, which if given in sufficient quantities, will be beneficial to the host organism. Studies on microorganisms are difficult to compare with each other because the same bacteria in different conditions can have different effects.

How is it possible to know if, concerning other bacteria, they do not act differently on the spot? It is impossible to do research and forecasts for all variants of microbiomes. But it is not even necessary to do so. The concept of a "symptom, a drug" should not be applied to micro-organisms as well. A shock to the microbiome is an expression of a disturbed cohabitation and is not a simple deficiency or an altered functioning of something.

Etymologically, "pro bios" means "in favor of life." Already a hundred years ago, Ilja Metchnikoff, the famous Russian doctor who won the Nobel Prize, stated: "Death resides in the intestine." He had discovered that the people of the Caucasus who ate daily products containing lactic acid (probiotics), were particularly healthy and resistant, as well as long-lived.

Today we know why! The intestine hosts the most sophisticated defense system in our body. It is where the immune cells are formed, which release the body from toxic substances, foreign bacteria, and viruses. A healthy bowel contains three times as many immune cells as in the spleen, bone marrow, and lymph nodes put together.

The immune cells fight to trigger our resistance, but they can only form in the intestine if a sufficient number of beneficial bacteria always correctly process the chyme, thus preventing fermentation or putrefaction processes from being activated. In a healthy individual, billions of intestinal bacteria work every day to ensure that digestion takes place regularly, and we feel good.

The two groups of bacteria, probiotics (good) and pathogens (bad) are in balance with each other, but the relationship can be unbalanced due to age, nutrition, acute intestinal diseases (diarrhea), chronic diseases (constipation) and antibiotic therapies. The use of natural supplements based on probiotic bacteria makes sense only if they are human-compatible and above all, if they are taken in a targeted manner for the compromised intestinal tract.

The probiotic bacteria make permanent colonies that last for 30/40 days, so it is useless to colonize continuously, on the contrary, it is better to gradually scale the intake of the bacteria up to a single or bi-weekly support. The replanting should be done twice a year at the change of season. It is vital, and for this reason, it is a question of restoring this coexistence of the microorganisms with each other and with all the epithelial cells. It can be done by eliminating the disturbing factors and strengthening the life force.

However, there is a particular need for suitable microorganisms that give a healthy boost to living together in the intestine. To get a cure, it is not enough to send any single laboratory-derived strains into the intestine to add to the hundreds or more of other species of microbes, so that they do what we have expected.

Everywhere on Earth, micro-organisms always live in a connected community. If this community is disturbed or destroyed, healing requires rebuilding of the community. By simply introducing single strains, perhaps the quantity of microbes is increased, but the necessary community is not yet reconstructed. Probiotics, impacts on anxiety, stress, and mental well-being to date; however, numerous studies show that the intestinal microbiome influences the brain, including emotions, thoughts, and perceptions.

According to the research in question, a good bacteria in fermented foods can increase the levels of a chemical in the brain called GABA, and it controls anxiety. GABA is a neurotransmitter that is imitated by many anti-anxiety drugs. In other words, including some fermented foods in your diet, each day may be the equivalent of taking a tablet to control anxiety.

As early as 1807, the French psychiatrist Phillipe Pinel said, "The main site of madness is generally in the region of the stomach and intestine." Pinel is known as the father of modern psychiatry and came to this quote after working with people with a mental health condition for many years. His words are finally starting to be researched and understood. In 2011 a team of Icelandic researchers carried out a study on mice to observe the effects of probiotics on stress and mood. To measure their stress level, the scientists put the guinea pigs in tanks full of water without the possibility of resting on the bottom. The idea was to compare the time spent swimming and thus the stress resistance of the two groups of mice: a first control group and a second group that had been given a bacterium, Lactobacillus rhamnosus, known for its beneficial effects on the 'intestine.

The mice of the second 37 group showed greater resistance and swam longer. Furthermore, their cortisol rate was minimal. The results of the experiment confirmed that probiotics could reduce stress while increasing resistance.

Another study carried out by Professor Stephen Collins, a gastroenterologist at the McMaster University in Hamilton (Canada) showed that the administration of probiotics to a mouse suffering from chronic intestinal inflammation could normalize brain behavior and activity. By treating inflammation with bacteria such as Bifidobacterium longum, it has been possible to reduce the level of stress and anxiety significantly. According to the study by Dinan, Stanton, Cryan (2013) some strains of lactobacilli and Bifidobacterium produce substances such as serotonin, acetylcholine and gamma-aminobutyric acid (GABA) that play an active role on the nervous system and our state mental. New research conducted in March 2016 validated these effects on humans. The results show that, in individuals between the ages of 20 and 55, probiotics

(Lactobacillus acidophilus, Lactobacillus casei and Bifidobacterium bifidum) continued for eight weeks to improve quality of life and alleviate symptoms of depression.

• **PREBIOTICS;** food for "good" bacteria when the microbiota is damaged by the frequent use of medicines, stress or the wrong diet, we need to introduce the most important bacterial strains for the intestine from the outside. And not just one, but different. The important thing is to take especially those microorganisms that can reach the small and large intestine and not eliminated as soon as they come into contact with gastric juices.

Nutrition allows the body's cells to provide the necessary nutrients, but also those intestinal bacteria need to live and grow. Depending on the types, some bacteria will grow more than others. The letter "prebiotic" means "before life" (prae-prima, bios-vita) but could also be translated as "food for bacteria." These substances help the good and useful bacteria "to become big and strong."

Prebiotics contribute to the development of a healthy and above all diverse intestinal microbiota, support its activity and favor the establishment of probiotics, i.e., beneficial bacteria. Often our good intestinal bacteria are undernourished, and on the contrary, we ingest foods that provide nutrition to pathogenic bacteria such as sugar or bad fats. Prebiotics are soluble vegetable fibers, nondigestible by humans, which serve as nourishment for the useful bacteria of the intestinal microbiota and which allow them to multiply, bringing benefits to the health of the host. Prebiotics are so called because they nourish the "probiotic" bacteria, literally "favorable to life."

The prebiotics are therefore indispensable for the maintenance of the microbiota, which will feed on these substances, transforming them into organic acids capable of performing protective actions on the intestinal mucosa.

• Important for weight control: The fibers increase in volume in the intestine, ensuring a rapid and persistent sense of satiety;

• Important in case of sluggish bowel: Increased volume fibers facilitate intestinal stool transit;

• Important in the presence of hemorrhoids and diverticula: The stools soften and can be excreted more easily;

• Important for well-being: The more bacteria are present in the intestine, the more energy is produced in our cells. This keeps you young and efficient. Soluble or prebiotic fibers are found mainly in the following foods;

• Ripe seasonal fruit rich in pectin's, such as apples, pears, oranges, grapefruit, strawberries, peaches, walnuts, bananas, prunes and dried figs

• Bulbs (garlic, onion);

• Radish or chicory roots;

• Vegetables such as Jerusalem artichokes, asparagus, crucifers, fennel, artichokes, beets, dandelion leaves, leeks, broccoli, beans, carrots, courgettes;

• Certain cereals or pseudocereals such as oats, rice, barley, rye, buckwheat;

• Legumes such as peas, lentils, chickpeas, white and red beans, soy;

• Seeds and mucilages like linseed, chia, psillo In particular Chicory root, chicory root is known mainly because of its similar taste to coffee, so much so that often people who cannot take caffeine use it just as an alternative to coffee. About half of the fibers contained in the chicory root are injected as a prebiotic fiber.

Insulin nourishes gut-friendly bacteria, improves digestion, and helps relieve constipation. It can also help to increase the production of bile, which in turn promotes the digestion of fats. The chicory root is also rich in antioxidant compounds that protect the liver from oxidative stress.

❖ Bananas, if green, bananas are also rich in resistant starch, which has important prebiotic effects. The banana also has a high content of tryptophan, a precursor of serotonin.

❖ Apple, the apple is rich in pectin, a polysaccharide with prebiotic properties. Specifically, it increases the amount of butyrate, a short-chain fatty acid that nourishes bacteria

Intestinal benefits and counteracts the development of harmful bacteria. Apples are also rich in polyphenols, antioxidant compounds found in many foods of plant origin. The combination of polyphenols and pectin helps improve digestive health and fat metabolism as well as reduce LDL cholesterol levels and decrease the risk of several cancers.

❖ Dandelion, Dandelion is usually used to prepare purifying teas. Dandelion leaves and flowers can be used as a salad. The fibers contained in the dandelion are mainly made up of inulin, which is useful for reducing constipation, promoting the health of good bacteria in the intestine, and strengthening the immune system. Dandelion is also known for its diuretic, anti-inflammatory, antioxidant, anti-cancer, and cholesterol-lowering properties.

❖ Artichoke: in addition to providing soluble and insoluble fiber, it is an excellent source of inulin, an important prebiotic. Inulin is, in fact, a soluble fiber that is not digested by intestinal enzymes.

❖ Topinambur, also known as Jerusalem artichoke or German turnip, has several benefits for human health. Some studies show that Jerusalem artichoke is useful for increasing the development of good bacteria in the colon, working even better than chicory root. Furthermore, this tuber helps to strengthen the immune system and prevent some metabolic disorders. Jerusalem artichoke is also rich in mineral salts such as potassium, phosphorus, iron, zinc, selenium, and magnesium. These nutrients promote the health of the nervous system and the muscular system.

❖ Garlic, onion, leek among the prebiotics present in garlic, onion, and leek we find inulin and fructooligosaccharides (or FOS). These plants belonging to the genus Allium are therefore excellent prebiotic foods, useful for the growth of Bifidobacterium in the intestine and to counteract the development of pathogenic bacteria. FOS improve intestinal microbiota, promote the breakdown of fats, and stimulate the immune system by increasing the production of nitric oxide in the cells. Also, garlic extract is effective in reducing the risk of heart disease and has antioxidant, anti-cancer, and antimicrobial properties. Garlic, onions, and leeks are also rich in quercetin, a flavonoid with antioxidant and anticancer properties. Furthermore, garlic, onion, and leek have natural antibiotic properties, bring benefits to the cardiovascular system, and counteract oxidative stress.

❖ Asparagus, contain a good supply of prebiotic inulin. Asparagus promotes a more balanced microbiota and also helps prevent some forms of cancer. In addition to the anti-cancer properties, the combination of fibers and antioxidants in asparagus makes this plant a good natural anti-inflammatory.

❖ Cocoa, cocoa beans is an excellent source of flavanols, which have prebiotic properties which are useful for the growth of healthy intestinal bacteria. Flavanols, moreover, favoring the production of nitric oxide, are beneficial for the heart and the whole cardiovascular system.

❖ Burdock root, most of the fibers contained in the burdock root are inulin and FOS. As already seen, inulin and FOS act as prebiotics, they can inhibit the growth of harmful bacteria in the intestine and improve the development of healthy microorganisms. At the same time, this prebiotics stimulates bowel movements and immune function. Burdock root also has 40 antioxidant and anti-inflammatory properties and helps to lower blood sugar levels.

❖ Barley and oats, barley and oats contain good amounts of beta-glucans and resistant starch. Beta-glucan is a prebiotic fiber that promotes the growth of good bacteria in the digestive system. The beta-glucans present in barley and oats can also decrease total LDL-related cholesterol, help lower blood glucose levels, and has significant anti-cancer effects. If oats are taken in the form of cereals, it is useful for slowing down digestion, thus being effective in increasing the sense of satiety and controlling hunger. Oats also have antioxidant and anti-inflammatory properties due to its phenolic acid content.

❖ Konjac root is very rich in fibers, of which almost half are represented by glucomannan, a highly viscous water-soluble polysaccharide. Glucomannan is a prebiotic food that is effective in promoting the growth of good colon bacteria, relieving constipation, and strengthening the immune system. Glucomannan can also reduce blood cholesterol, help lose weight, and improve carbohydrate metabolism.

❖ Linseed, flaxseed fibers are useful for the development of probiotics and to regulate intestinal peristalsis, while reducing the amount of fat absorbed. Thanks to their content of phenolic compounds, flax seeds also have antioxidant and anti-cancer properties and also help to regulate blood sugar levels.

❖ Algae, marine algae represent a great source of prebiotics. About 50-85% of the algae fiber content is soluble fiber. Studies have shown that algae can provide many health benefits. They promote the growth of good bacteria in the intestine, prevent the proliferation of harmful microorganisms, increase immune function, and reduce the risk of colon cancer.

❖ the root of yacón, the prebiotics mainly present in this tuber are the fructooligosaccharides (FOS) and inulin. Yacón prebiotics can improve the development of intestinal bacteria, reduce constipation, stimulate the immune system, promote the absorption of mineral salts, and regulate fat levels in the blood. Yacón also contains phenolic compounds which give this vegetable antioxidant property.

❖ Jicama root, the jicama, or Mexican potato, is a tuber that contains very few calories but many fibers, including inulin. Jicama root helps improve digestive health, insulin sensitivity, blood glucose levels, and immune defenses. The fruits of the plant are also an excellent source of all essential amino acids.

❖ Wheat bran, it is the outer layer of wheat grain. It is an excellent source of prebiotics. It also contains a special type of fiber known as arabinoxylan oligosaccharides (AXOS). AXOS fibers account for more than half of the fiber content of wheat bran. The AXOS fiber of wheat bran is effective in increasing the presence of Bifidobacterium in the intestine. Wheat bran is also useful for reducing digestive problems such as flatulence, stomach cramps, and abdominal pain. AXOS-rich cereals also have antioxidant and anti-cancer effects. 68 Prebiotics Inulin + Fructose Fermentation by MI (action of colon bacteria) Production of short chain fatty acids (propionic, butyric and acetic acid)

• Growth of "good" bacteria

• Lowering of intestinal pH (acidification) or Decrease of harmful bacteria

• Improvement of intestinal wall mucus or Good selectivity of the mucosa

• Reduction of inflammation.

Chapter 6

FEEDING BACTERIAL GROUP

The different bacterial composition depends on genetic, food, geographical, or age-related factors. Moreover, it undergoes constant modifications throughout life. Each has a peculiar microbiota in terms of bacterial species composition. Somehow a unique bacterial barcode. Just as we have our blood group, in the same way, we would belong to a specific "bacterial group," also called "enterotype." The main ones would be three: bacteroid, ruminococcus, prevotella, and the likelihood of belonging to either of them would depend on the predominant bacterial species in our intestine. Unlike the genetically determined blood type, the belonging enterotype is closely related to the type of diet.

According to the study conducted by James Lewis' team at the Perelman School of Medicine in Philadelphia (Pennsylvania) which shows that belonging to an enterotype would not depend on either the age or the geographical origin of the individual, but on his / her diet. A diet rich in meat and animal fats would lead to the bacterial type, the most frequent, while a carbohydrate-based diet would favor Prevotella. The diet, therefore, determines the individual bacterial profile, which in turn affects the personality, behavior, and mental balance of the person. A microbiome needs: - a diet adapted to the species - a healthy lifestyle - the introduction of life-promoting bacteria

The natural supply of the intestine with bacteria occurs through the microbes present in food and through the colonization of the environment in which we live. The most important criteria for an adequate microbiome diet are the content of dietary fiber, the composition, and quality of food, their bacterial content, and the fact that they are free of poisons. Feeding should be as fresh and natural as possible. The more modified a plant or animal product is, the more they are far from the natural conditions of the intestine. The only exception among these is microbiologically fermented foods. Since the components of the diet should adapt to the digestive enzymes of all the cells of the intestine as a key in the lock, each step of technical processing hides the risk of a discrepancy.

The parts of foods that cannot be well digested stimulate the growth of bacteria that break down, whose metabolic products disturb more than they feed on it. For this reason, nutrition must also be as close to nature as possible. During growth, plants absorb free bacteria and genes through the roots, such as bacterial plasmids, which we eat as part of a natural cycle.

The consequences of any soil processing, therefore, come into our body. We cannot be healthier than the soil on which our foods grow. Every poison in food, even if only in a quantum way, is not limited to acting alone, but requires a splitting or transformation by bacteria. The toxic substances that are released from these processes can kill bacteria, damage intestinal cells, weaken the microbiome, and be absorbed into the body. Poisons in the intestine can render enzymes ineffective, disrupt the bacterial metabolic passages and damage digestion. Parts of the materials also belong to the packaging of the poison, such as chemical softeners in plastic films and aluminum. It is evident that dietary fibers have an existential role in microbiome nutrition. Through an adequate diet that is rich in fiber, it will be easy to promote the growth rate and the composition of bacteria and the health of the microbiome.

The consumption of fresh spices has a boost on intestinal bacteria and manages to regulate them in a multifaceted manner. Anise, cumin, pepper, garlic, marjoram, cinnamon, curry, cloves or rosemary have a modeling action on bacteria, yeasts and molds are decidedly antimicrobial concerning unwanted single-celled organisms. Cinnamon, basil, rosemary, and sage, for example, contain camphor. Many spices contain essential oils which, as is known, inhibit bacterial growth.

When humans still personally fed from the labor of the fields, the bacterial composition was linked to the types present in the farmstead, in the barn and the vegetable garden, and the bacterial flora that was assumed was all the more colorful, the more diverse it was the organic whole of the farmhouse with cows, chickens, sheep, pigs, oxen and donkeys, orchards, vegetable gardens, dogs and cats. Such a variety has a stabilizing action on the microbiome, and this is why the health of people living in the countryside is better. In modern food there are too few bacteria, to remedy this there are three possibilities:

- Grow your food

- Ingest healthy bacteria with food

- Consume fermented foods

THE IMPORTANCE OF FERMENTED FOOD

Fermented foods have a multi-millennial tradition and have already served our ancestors as a supply of fresh bacteria during the winter when it was almost impossible to introduce them with fresh fruit and vegetables.

Bacterial fermentation opens food, bacterial enzymes transform raw materials and release cellular components that are in turn digested bacteriologically. Derived compounds, including these vitamins and micronutrients, are particularly favorable for the health of the intestine and therefore for the health of the whole body. In the meantime, it is known that the bioactive substances that derive from it modulate the immune system, regulate the rate of blood sugar, and slow down inflammation.

In sauerkraut lactic acid bacteria, yeasts and other microbes ferment white cabbage in fatty acids and large amounts of ascorbic acid (vitamin C). The formation of acids prevents the growth of mold and from the microbes of putrefaction, and this derives long conservation.

Only in fermented foods is there a long shelf life accompanied by a healthy bacterial intake. Lactic acid bacteria, but not yeasts, can penetrate inside some vegetables, such as cucumbers, and transform carbohydrates on the spot into more easily digestible compounds.

If you compare the microbiome of people, who consume many fermented foods with that of those who have different eating habits, in the first one, there are more common bacterial strains for these foods. Consequently, it can be concluded that the 45 fermented foods have a direct influence on the composition of the microbiome.

In some studies, it was found that subjects who had consumed fermented rice starch, fatigue, and susceptibility to stress decreased compared to the control group. Neurotransmitters were activated in their brains that reduced fears. In our consumer society, in reality, fermented foods are rarely present on our tables either because they require time for preparation, or because we are used to always eating the same things. We are not used to creating live enzymes in the home, probiotics that our bodies desperately need.

The correlation between healthy bacteria in our body and physical health or emotional health is instead very interdependent. Fermented foods and beverages are a source of ancient health that has been lost over the years. Before the introduction of the refrigeration system, food traditions had to preserve their vegetables and dairy products exclusively through 'lacto-fermentation' processes, processes that enriched the content and nutritional value of the products consumed, in a significant way too.

Fermentation involves generation of the appropriate circumstances in which natural organisms thrive and reproduce. These are ancient rituals that humans have practiced for many generations. They are an important link to the world of natural medicine and to our ancestors, whose intelligent observations allow us to enjoy the benefits of these transformations still.

The use of these foods is a way of also incorporating the "wild" in our body, and becoming one with the natural world. It is a bit like entering an alchemical relationship with bacteria and fungi and bringing naturally prepared food and drinks to our tables. By eating a good variety of fermented foods, we can promote the diversity of microbial cultures in our body.

Biodiversity, now increasingly seen as an essential factor for the survival of large-scale ecosystems, it is also recognized for minor ecosystems. Our body is a micro-ecosystem that can work more effectively once populated by many varieties of microorganisms.

By fermenting foods and beverages with microorganisms present in our family environment, we become more connected with the vital forces of the world around us. Our environment becomes ourselves, as we invite the microbial populations with which we share the environment to enter our diet and our intestinal ecology.

Fermentation is the opposite of homogenization and uniformity. The do-it-yourself fermentation rediscovers and reinterprets the vast fermentation techniques used by our ancestors, and develops the ecological culture of our body based on how we honor the vital forces around us. Sandor Katz likes to define it as a "science," and the basis of human culture.

It is fascinating to think that similar conservation procedures can be found in popular traditions in the most diverse places on earth and unfortunately, these are in danger of extinction, since man surrounded by the products of large retailers, has lost contact with the real food of the past.

The preserves that are found in the supermarket have very little to do with the ones I'm talking about, being almost certainly sterilized at high temperatures without being fermented, and immersed in vinegar with maybe artificial preservatives, the result of which is a scarce food nutritional value, if not sugars and vegetable fibers.

When food passes through the fermentation process, it begins to produce beneficial bacteria, lactobacilli, which support the health of our body, along with other "good" bacterial strains. Without a fair amount of these healthy bacteria in our body, we begin to have symptoms such as depression, anxiety, ADHD, allergies, asthma, digestive problems, skin problems, and more.

Lacto-fermentation doesn't only allow us to preserve the nutrients present in the food longer, but also to enrich foods with new nutritional qualities. Let's take the sauerkraut example: once fermented, cabbage contains more vitamin C than raw vegetables.

The bacteria responsible for fermentation, the lactobacilli, synthesize vitamins B and C. Many dissertations on fermented vegetables states the fact that Captain Cook was able to keep the scurvy on his ships at bay by forcing the sailors to consume sauerkraut: the device worked, as we now know, because fermentation increases the content of vitamin C in cabbage. We also know that it increases the quality of other vitamins and minerals. Moreover, thanks to lacto fermentation, foods are "predigested," thus increasing their digestibility and bioavailability. With this method, lipids are already transformed into fatty acids, amino acid proteins, and starch into glucose and maltose.

These essential "bricks," the nutrients, will be assimilated without having to be digested. It also enriches foods with beneficial lactic ferments. Also, the acidification of the food obtained with lacto fermentation causes a slight increase in the degree of acidity in the intestine, thus preventing the development of pathogenic genes. A lactofermentated food is a "live" food, rich in enzymes and microorganisms, and therefore has a high vital charge. When you start consuming fermented foods daily, you feed the body with a nice battery of probiotics, vitamins, and live enzymes.

Eating fermented foods allows several benefits, including:

• Help remove toxins from the body.

• Strengthen the immune system. 47

• Improve digestion.

• Absorb and use nutrients to the fullest.

• Strengthen the immune system and fight inflammation.

• Combat candida albicans.

• Increase the energy levels of our body.

• Balance hormones.

Fermentation to preserve food and improve its nutritional qualities has been used for thousands of years, and indeed in nature, it has been used for billions of years, stopping it is impossible. The consumption of fermented foods contributes to creating a healthy ecosystem within the organism that improves the overall balance and prevents disease.

Yin fermentation, which occurs in foods preserved in salt, yang is bearable acidification because it is moderated by salt and pressure. Storage in vinegar (yin) causes corrosion, and it is good for more yang meat like game. Our life is inevitably linked to the life of microbes; fermented foods thus constitute both a food and a remedy. However, it has been possible to demonstrate the existence of an annual microbiome rhythm. The fact that bacteria are stimulated to double through food intake and then return to their original number can also be considered a rhythm.

A recent Swedish study conducted on about six thousand women has shown how the weakening of bones and in particular fractures, such as those of the hip, diminish by combining fermented foods with fruits and vegetables. As Dr. Claudio Pagano, specialist in Endocrinology and Metabolic Diseases and Associate Professor of Internal Medicine at the University of Padua, explains: "According to this study in post-menopausal women, it would, therefore, be preferable to take calcium through the products at fermented milk base rather than simple milk because they are poorer in pro-oxidant substances".

For decades, an American doctor, Dr. McBride has successfully treated adults and children with serious illnesses, including autism, epilepsy, mood disorders, arthritis, multiple sclerosis, celiac disease, and many others, with its GAPS protocol. A key component of the GAPS program is the daily consumption of fermented foods. Fermented foods, besides being powerful chelators (detoxifier), contain much higher levels of probiotics than probiotic supplements, which makes them ideal for optimizing intestinal microflora.

In addition to helping to break down and eliminate heavy metals and other toxins from the body, beneficial intestinal bacteria perform as I have already said, a series of amazing functions. The GAPS nutritional protocol aims to restore the integrity of the lining of the intestine. Its dietary component consists of easily digestible and dense foods in nutrition, including fermented foods. A group of researchers from the College of William and Mary collaborated with the University of Maryland. They are tested more than 700 students. The results, published in the journal Psychiatry Research, showed that eating fermented foods relieves anxiety and neurosis. In particular, those who ate fermented foods, including pickles, sauerkraut and yogurt were stronger psychically, and adding a small amount of fermented food to each meal will save money because they can contain 100 times more probiotics than a supplement!

Natural variety of microflora. As long as the fermented and cultured food you eat is varied, you will get a much wider variety of beneficial bacteria than you can get from a supplement. Here from last, a compelling reason to start fermenting: The fermentation, even before doing well for health, creates perfect things. Let's open a jar and let's get lost in the smells and the new, engaging, unique flavors of fermentation.

THE "CORE MICROBIOTA" FOR THE LONGEVITY

By influencing multiple aspects of human physiology, such as the proper functioning of the immune system and energy metabolism, the intestinal microbiota can represent an essential part in defining how much a human being can age while keeping himself in good health. Several published studies investigate the relationship between specific bacterial strains present in our intestines and longevity.

Populations with a diet made up of large quantities of fermented foods are those with slower brain aging. But is there a connection between intestinal microbiota and life expectancy? This conclusion was reached by all-Italian research recently published in the international journal "Current Biology," which investigated the composition of the microbiota in subjects of very different age groups.

It is the first study in the world to analyze the intestinal microbiota of exceptionally long-lived people over the age of one hundred. The research was conducted by a group of microbial ecology experts on the health of the Department of Pharmacy and Biotechnology, and by the research group on studies on aging and longevity of the Department of Specialized, Diagnostic and Experimental Medicine of the University of Bologna, with the partnership of the Institute of Biomedical Technologies of the National Research Council (ITB-CNR) of Milan. Scholars have analyzed, in particular, the microbiota of semi and supercentenarian subjects between the ages of 105 and 110, comparing it with that of centenarians between the ages of 99 and 104, with that of seniors aged 65-75 and of adults between the ages of 20 and 50, all enrolled in the same geographical area to limit the differences due to eating habits and lifestyle. "Longevity - explained researcher UniBo, Elena Biagi - is a complex trait in which genetics, the environment, and chance play a key role.

By influencing multiple aspects of human physiology, such as the proper functioning of the immune system and energy metabolism, the intestinal microbiota can represent an essential element in defining how and how much a human being can age while keeping himself in good health". The research revealed the existence of a "core microbiota": a sort of "fixed" portion of the intestinal ecosystem composed mainly of species of microorganisms belonging to the families Ruminococcaceae,

Lachnospiraceae, and Bacteroidaceae, generally associated with the state of health and producers of molecules beneficial for our body, such as SCFA (short chain fatty acids).

The research confirms that with the advancing age, the overall abundance of these species within the intestinal microbiota decreases, favoring the proliferation of other species of microorganisms, present in low percentage in young adults. Furthermore, in aging the relationship of co-occurrence between microbial species not belonging to the "core," i.e., the frequency with which two species appear together in an individual's intestinal microbiota. "These typical features of an ecosystem associated with an aging organism are maintained in the intestinal microbiota of long-lived and extremely long-lived 50 individuals.

At the same time, however, the intestinal microbiota of the semi-supercenters shows signs of a parallel proliferation of anti-inflammatory, immunomodulatory micro-organisms and promoters of intestinal epithelial health, such as Bifidobacterium and Akkermansia ".

Ancient food traditions around the world have kept the use of fermented foods and beverages in almost every meal and therefore do not suffer particularly from digestive problems, autoimmune problems, and emotional problems, which are the major afflictions of the modern world.

Primitive and traditional diets maintain in their habits foods with a high content of enzymes and beneficial bacteria taken from vegetables, fruits, beverages, dairy products, and fermented condiments. The connection point between emotions and eating behavior is a neurotrophic stimulating factor present in the brain - brain-derived neurotrophic factor or BDNF - which is linked to cognitive aging: this BDNF is influenced by the microbiome.

Chapter 7

YOU ARE WHAT YOU EAT WHEN YOU TAKE ACCOUNT OF YOUR INTESTINAL MICROBES

The amount of food we consume is controlled by three systems that interact closely: in addition to the control of appetite regulated by the hypothalamus, the other two that play an essential role are the dopamine reward circuit and the executive control system located in the prefrontal cortex which, if necessary, can voluntarily overlap with all other control systems. In the world of hunter-gatherers, which is characterized by limited food reserves and high energy demands, the urge to eat was driven by the constant existential need for food.

This basic system for assessing caloric needs was assisted by the reward circuit, which provided the impetus and motivation for finding food. The nerves containing dopamine, which include large portions of the brain's reward network, promise us a substantial reward if we perform a certain action, and have a leading role in modulating the justification and sustainability of the behaviors necessary to obtain the reward, in this case, the stimulus and the motivation to go in search of food.

Millions of years of evolution have optimized this complicated interaction between reward and appetite for a world of limited and difficult to obtain food reserves. However, this programming of our brain systems linked to food intake loses much of its adaptive value in the world in which most of us live today.

In a modern industrialized society, with access to highly desirable foods and with reduced levels of physical activity, the stimulus of the reward circuit can easily overwhelm the control system that calculates our daily caloric needs, and it is often necessary to intervene voluntarily to avoid to overreact and gain weight.

One of the behaviors that can result from this remodeling of appetite control mechanisms is food addiction. There is recent evidence to suggest that an unlimited activity of the reward circuit in food-dependent individuals could further compromise bowel function. In a recent study on alcohol-dependent individuals, it was shown that the desire for alcohol during periods of abstinence was positively correlated with the intestinal permeability of the individuals themselves and changes in their intestinal microbiota. The idea that our intestinal microbes can influence the reward circuit and play a role in food addiction has inspired many hypotheses about the relationship between ourselves and the intestinal microbiome, even questioning the idea of voluntariness.

In a provocative article, Joe Alcock, a lecturer at the University of Mexico, recently suggested that intestinal microbes may be subjected to strong selective pressure to manipulate human eating behavior in ways that increase their health, sometimes at the expense of ours. Intestinal microbes can do this through two potential interactive strategies.

On the one hand, taking over the dopamine-controlled reward circuit could generate desires for some particular foods in whose consumption they have specialized and which give them an advantage over other competing microbial species. Secondly, they could create negative moods, for example, by making us feel depressed, which remain until we eat some components of the foods that benefit these intestinal microbes.

The impulse to consume the so-called comparison foods and the concept of food addiction are both excellent examples of behaviors that are partially manipulated by some types of intestinal microbiota to obtain the preferred substances.

Equally drastic changes are taking place in the differentiation of microorganisms that live in the soil, in the rapidly declining microbiota of bees and butterflies, and in the microbes that live in our gastrointestinal tract. An important question is whether this double chemical insult to the natural ecosystem of the environment (from which our food comes) and the internal ones of intestinal microbes (which play a key role in the brain's health) of our farm animals and ourselves are contributing to the dramatic increase of some brain diseases during of the last fifty years. Emulsifiers are detergent-like molecules that help mix two liquids that do not combine easily, such as oil and water.

These detergent-like molecules have a negative aspect, as they are able to alter the protective mucus layer that covers the inner surface of the gastrointestinal tract, providing microbes with easier access to the intestinal walls, and thus allowing intestinal microbes to pass through it and gain access to nearby immune cells, favoring the so-called metabolic toxemia. In addition to the dangers to our metabolic health of the commonly used food additives, there are significant implications for the functioning of the gut-microbiome-brain axis and our brain health. Food emulsifiers just like animal fats and artificial sweeteners can alter the profile of our microbiota in a way that can promote the development of low-intensity inflammation in the intestine, in other organs, and the brain, including the areas that they control the appetite.

An excessive amount of similar ingredients exposes us to excessive consumption of high-calorie foods, which would only aggravate the inflammation and worsen the situation.

A look at the "useful" bacteria

The Akkermansia municiphila lives in the mucosa that protects the intestinal cells, to which it can attach itself. The bacterium activates genes that increase the combustion of fats and also has a strange predilection for the mucosa, from which the name "muciphila" is derived, which roughly means "who loves the mucosa." The germ willingly demolishes the mucous layer of the intestine and eats it. It renews the intestine, removes the old mucosa, stimulating the calceiform cells to produce new and fresh ones.

Today, it is well known that these microorganisms play an essential role in maintaining the barrier function exerted by the intestine. Bifidobacterium have always accompanied us and are present in good numbers in the intestines of newborns, especially those breastfed, they make premature babies grow better and keep children thin. They are present in greater numbers in lean people, while in those who are overweight sometimes there is no trace. Pregnant women gain less weight if they take good amounts of these beneficial bacteria.

The Firmicutes, bacteria present in the large intestine could be defined as "waste users." Above all, the nutrients that are not transformed in the small intestine break down and digest. The strength of the Firmicutes lies precisely in the fact that they exploit the parts of food that are difficult to digest and can make extra portions of fatty acids available to the body. They get more energy than others, even from low-calorie foods.

This species of bacteria are often present not only in people who have to struggle with extra pounds but also as scholars from California and Arizona have recently observed, in the inhabitants of the colder regions. There are 54 "bacteria of the dawn of time," in times of famine; these bacteria were beneficial because they manage to get more calories from food, favoring the formation of fat deposits.

Faced with the same dish, it is the intestinal microbiota that decides how many calories the body has to absorb and transform into fatty tissue, and if we get up from the table satisfied or still hungry, then, the caloric tables are not worth it, because its body derives from every single carrot or leaf of salad much more energy than the norm.

Ruminococcus bromii typically triggers the disintegration of resistant starch, and this so-called starch is contained in a wide variety of plant-based foods, including bananas, potatoes, seeds, legumes, and unrefined whole grains. In most individuals, resistant starch is completely fermented and transformed into short-chain fatty acids in the colon, but this ability is lacking in the intestinal microbiota of some individuals.

This bacterium makes the partially digested substrate available to other bacteria, which then further break down the individual sugars using different enzymes. These bacteria play a key role, as they carry out activities that are essential for the optimal functioning of the ecosystem as a whole.

In the intestinal microbiota, if an important species such as Ruminococcus bromii is reduced or absent, the ability of all other microbes to carry out their work (such as metabolizing complex carbohydrates) is compromised on the contrary if one of the related species is absent, promptly another will take over to do his job.

Chapter 8
THE INTESTINAL MICROBIOTA AND OBESITY

With a good quantity bacteria composition, it is possible to extract caloric energy from the dietary fiber for the body and protect it, simultaneously. It is not just the quantity of what we eat that determines our energy supply, but rather how our microbiome can exploit this quantity. The caloric content of food is usually calculated using standard conversion tables, so it is believed that every gram of carbohydrate provides four calories, every gram of nine fat calories and so on. These tables present the calories of food as a fixed value.

Peter Turnbaugh's work suggests instead that the matter is not so linear. If microbes are at our service to extract energy from food, it is our particular community of microbes that determines how many calories we get from what we eat, not a standard conversion table. Obesity is rather a dysfunction of the body's energy storage system.

The particular series of microbes that we host determines our ability to extract energy from food. After the small intestine has digested and absorbed everything it can from what we ate, the remains move into the large intestine, where most of our microbes live. Here they work as factory workers, each splitting the preferred molecules and absorbing what it succeeds. The rest is reduced to a form quite simple to be absorbed through the lining of the large intestine.

The diet of each of us affects the strains we host. To understand how the diet acts on the microbiota, I have to illustrate once again their dynamic coexistence. Microorganisms multiply depending on the environment in which they live, for example, from the food we eat.

Bacteria are everywhere, and the number of microorganisms involved in the path of food in the intestinal tract increases continuously.

After being tasted, mixed with saliva and chewed, each morsel ends up in the esophagus and from there into the stomach, where so far 120 different bacterial strains have been found, and where the gastric juices act on the chyme. And here it rests first. It is mixed with hydrochloric acid, numerous enzymes capable of breaking down proteins and a few others capable of breaking down lipids, bacteria and their metabolic products. The distribution of the juices is regulated by the hormones that form in the mucous membrane of the stomach and which are related to the small intestine, the pancreas, and the vagus nerve. There are also effects of bowel feedback.

For example, if there are many fats and simple sugars in the intestine, a greater quantity of GIP hormone is released into the blood. This leads to the distribution of insulin and, if this occurs in unnaturally high doses, inhibits stomach movements and the production of gastric juices. The food remains in the stomach as long as the juices that are acting in it have not decomposed the contents to such an extent that the small intestine can continue digesting them. When it comes out of the stomach, the food is neutralized and through the pylorus pushed, in small portions, towards the duodenum. All along the digestive tract, the food, passing from one organ to another, encounters lymphatic tissues that react to its contact but also with the bacteria that are found there.

Food compounds that are broken down by the microbiome act on the blood cells of the body and from here regulate the enzymatic steps and the hormonal balance as soon as the food reaches the digestive organs, the bacteria that conform to the incoming food multiply, managing to double within 20-40 min. For sugars, the microbes that digest sugars are multiplied, for fats those that digest fats, for proteins those that digest proteins, for each component there are suitable microbes, there are also the most flexible ones.

Congratulations to those who have an effective team in their stomach where all the necessary microbes are present. This explains why an impoverishment of bacterial strains always implies lower tolerability and flexibility concerning food. Our microbial network is like the keyboard of a piano playing on our foods.

Depending on the needs, the composition changes rapidly. During an experiment, some volunteers consumed food of exclusively vegetable or animal origin for five days respectively. In this study published in "Nature," it was found that one day after abandoning the normal diet for one exclusively based on cereals, fruit, vegetables, legumes or exclusively based on meat, eggs, and cheese the bacterial strains in the microbiome they had adjusted to the changes by changing their community.

Two days after returning to a normal diet, the microbiome also returned to its previous condition. The thing that caught the eye in all this was that the diet based on products of animal origin had a much stronger effect than a vegetable diet and that it was possible to find the microorganisms present in food in the intestine. To the extent that the food has moved away from its natural origin, i.e., the plants, it has also moved away from the characteristics of our microbiome. The food of today and the intestinal community, dating back more than thousands of years ago, suddenly no longer agree. In the archaeological stool tests, a microbiome similar to the one found today in people belonging to cultures that traditionally live in the countryside was found.

The more a diet moves away from the natural light of the sun and the soil, factors that have helped a plant to grow, the more it consumes its original microbiome. Each meal we take, therefore forms a certain mix of bacteria in the intestine that corresponds to its composition. And every diet potentially stimulates a particular mix, but this only happens if the microbes that could multiply with a certain diet are still present and find the living conditions in which they can thrive. Among these are the value of the Ph., the dietary fibers, the culture media, and microbial partners with which they are linked in a metabolic team. If something is missing, a given diet may not have the effect it would otherwise have. For this reason, every sensible diet must also be accompanied by a bacterial supply. Every type of diet inevitably involves a certain kind of influence on the microbiota. Likewise, a targeted dietary composition can make a real miracle and free a person from extra pounds of weight and disease. It is true that the same diet can, however, not have any effect on another subject. This depends on the condition of the microbiota. For example, a bowel can make us understand what kind of bacterial supply the body needs. If you are craving pickled pickles or herring, this may indicate a need for lactic acid bacteria. On the other hand, if you want apricot or dried fruit, you may lack magnesium. If, on the other hand, sardines in oil and gruyere are sought, a need for calcium is indicated. The nature that feeds us and the food we put on the table have little in common. In every process of technical elaboration every food loses its content, energy, and naturalness. During the grinding, white flour-based products lose most of their micronutrients, such as selenium, zinc, B-group vitamins.

In a study that analyzed the influence of a different diet in children in Italy and Burkina Faso, it was found that in both groups' representatives of each of the four major intestinal bacterial strains were found in the intestine, but in African children, the Actinobacteria and Bacteroidetes prevailed in European children Firmicutes and Proteobacteria.

The researchers attributed this to the high proportion of plant fibers in the African diet. This also allowed African children to extract from food, thanks to bacteria, enough vital energy with less caloric intake than in Europe. More energy with less food.

Catia Sternini, a UCLA neuroscientist expert in the enteric nervous system, stated that some intestinal taste receptors may react to the 58 metabolites produced by the gut microbiota and that their alterations due to high fat intake and related changes in this complex of microorganisms could play a role in obesity.

Perhaps the microbiota could represent the missing link between the intake and consumption of calories? Patrice Cani, a professor of nutrition and metabolism in Belgium, identified that when skinny men stored energy, they produced more fat cells, filling each with a small amount of fat. In the obese, on the contrary, this healthy energy storage process did not occur. Instead of producing more fat cells, they produced larger ones and filled them with increasing amounts of fat.

According to Cani, inflammation, and the lack of new fat cells were a sign that overweight subjects had overstepped the healthy energy storage process. Dogs suspected that the "obese" microbiota caused inflammation and change in fat accumulation. He knew that some of the bacteria that live in the intestine were coated with a molecule called lipopolysaccharide or LPS, which if it entered the blood acted as a toxin.

Among the microbes present in different quantities in the intestine of the obese and lean is a species called Akkermansia muciniphila. This bacterium is linked to weight: the less Akkermansia, an individual, possesses the higher is his BMI. About 4% of the microbial community of lean individuals belongs to this species, while in the obese it is almost absent. It lives as the name suggests, on the surface of the thick layer of mucus that covers the inner wall of the intestine (muciniphila means "lover of the mucus").

This mucus forms a barrier that prevents the microbiota from passing into the blood, where it could do damage. The amount of Akkermansia that individuals possess is not only related to their BMI: the lower the proportion of this bacterium, the thinner the mucus layer and the more LPs are present in the blood.

It may seem that Akkermansia is common in the intestines of thin people because it benefits from that thick layer of mucus, but in reality, its job is to convince the intestinal lining cells to produce more. The Akkermansia sends a chemical request that activates the human mucus-producing genes, thus providing a home for itself and preventing LPS from passing into the blood. In 2015, a group of researchers from the Institut de la Santé et de la Recherché Medicale (Inserm) in Rouen showed that our feelings of hunger and satiety are directly linked to the needs of our intestinal bacteria. The intestinal bacteria would, therefore, have some control over their host's sense of hunger and satiety. This opens up interesting perspectives about the treatment of obesity and its link with the microbiota. To develop, the intestinal bacteria would also push us to choose the best foods for them.

Chapter 9

MICROBIOTA AND MENTAL WELL-BEING

There is a new scientific evidence that underlying gastrointestinal problems, allergies, autoimmune diseases, and even obesity are disorders of bodily microbes. And it's not just the physical health that is affected, but also the mental health, from anxiety to depression, from obsessive-compulsive disorder to autism. With the help of new research on the microbiome, it was suddenly recognized that in the understanding between the intestine and the nervous system bacteria have something important to say, they are fundamental for our psychic abilities, our thinking, our feelings, and our will.

It has already been discovered that certain intestinal bacteria are missing or predominant in mental illnesses. Attention deficit syndrome, hyperactivity, Alzheimer's, multiple sclerosis can be explained as diseases of the microbiome.

Many disorders are caused by the fact that we could not adequately take care of the old extension of human cells: our microbes. It is essential to restore the entire subtly woven cooperative structure into the intestine. And this involves an even more compact dimension, namely that of the relations of intestinal bacteria with our psyche and our brain. Neurodegenerative disorders are also on the rise. In industrialized countries, one person in 100 has Parkinson's disease, and in the United States, at least half a million suffer from it, with around 50,000 new cases diagnosed each year.

It has been estimated that the number of Parkinson's cases will double by 2030. Recent research shows that the enteric nervous system undergoes typical Parkinson's degeneration long before the appearance of the classic symptoms of the disease and that this is accompanied by alterations in the intestinal microbial composition of patients. Recent evidence is beginning to link some of the most devastating brain diseases and the most common neuro intestinal pathologies to alterations in how the gut microbes communicate with the brain, and the effects on the relationship of our lifestyle and diet.

From a 2018 study, researchers also observed a significant negative association between depression levels and the number of bacterial species observed, which means that higher levels of depression were associated with lower diversity of microbiomes. Nature Reviews Neuroscience has recently hosted an extensive review, written by two researchers from the psychiatry department of the Irish University of Cork, on the "Impact of the microbiota on the brain and behavior." directions, in the sense that they influence each other, for better or for worse. For example, a condition of emotional stress alters the composition of the microbiota and, in turn, a condition of inflammatory bowel stress alters brain activity. With what mechanisms? The effects of brain stress are mediated by the release of cortisol, adrenaline, and noradrenaline which modify the balance between bacterial strains and the local immune system; at the same time, stress hormones make the intestinal barrier more permeable to the pathogenic strains present in the mucosa which then move into the intestine. In the opposite direction, an alteration of the intestinal microbiota determines the release of inflammatory cytokines which, traveling with the vagus nerve and blood, reach the brain. The verification of the correctness of this reasoning also comes from experimental and clinical studies. A work just published in the specialized journal "Cell" by Sarkis K. Mazmanian and eleven collaborators of the California Institute of Technology, highlighted the interactions between the microbiome and cognitive behavioral disorders. It was already known that, in humans, disorders of nervous and behavioral development, including the diagnostic spectrum of autism, are often accompanied by gastrointestinal disorders, sometimes even serious ones. Mazamanian and colleagues wanted to see more clearly and have to conduct the study with a mouse. In essence, observing the alterations of the gastrointestinal microbiome in mothers and then introducing into the offspring a bacterium present in man (called Bacteroides fragilis) which modifies intestinal permeability and ecology, have achieved improvements in pre-existing defects of communicative behavior, greater resistance to stress, fewer symptoms of anxiety and better success in motor skills and sensitivity.

The introduction of this microorganism has radically altered various components of the metabolism, thanks to the ability these bacteria have to produce substances necessary for the organism that hosts them.

Other refined experiments, with sterile mice and with targeted insertions of these microorganisms, have confirmed the impact that intestinal metabolism has on the brain and behavior. These scholars conclude that there exists, at least in the mouse, an intestine-brain axis that is mediated by the microbiome and has clear consequences on syndromes that reproduce the spectrum of autistic disorders. The consequences of the alteration of the gut-brain-microbiota dialogue could occur very late in life when both the diversity and the ability to recover the intestinal microbiota decrease.

This probably makes us more vulnerable to the development of degenerative brain disorders such as Alzheimer's or Parkinson's. To prevent these devastating pathologies, we must pay attention to how we treat our gut-brain-microbiota axis well in advance, well before brain damage occurs with severe symptoms.

With the new knowledge on the intestine and after recognizing the importance of the enteric nervous system, it was established that even before it occurs in the brain of the head, degenerative changes appear in the intestinal brain. Swallowing problems, slowed stomach emptying, intestinal constipation can be early signs of Parkinson's disease. Some cells of the enteric nervous system begin to degenerate years before the other symptoms of Parkinson appear, compromising the elaborate functioning of the second brain, slowing down the peristalsis and the transit of the feces through the colon.

The intestinal microbiota undergoes major changes in Parkinson's patients as demonstrated by a recent study by Filip Scheperjans, of the University of Helsinki. The team found that the microbiota of Parkinson's patients had reduced levels of prevotella bacteria, compared to the microbiota of healthy people.

The prevotella bacterium thrives in the intestines of people on a plant-based diet and is reduced in people who eat fewer vegetables and more meat, milk, and derivatives. Although other factors are also fundamental, such as genetic vulnerability or other environmental toxins, several other types of studies offer evidence to support the hypothesis that this disease may also affect the intestine-brain-microbial axis.

A vegetarian diet that modifies the microbiome, for example, reduces the risk of contracting Parkinson's. And we know that intestinal microbial diversity decreases in old age, at a time in life when the intestinal microbiome becomes more vulnerable to disorders. Perhaps not by chance, Parkinson's creeps in around sixty years. It has also been observed for some time that people with mental illness always have a disturbed intestinal function. Constipation, diarrhea, irritable bowel, intolerances, and inflammatory bowel diseases are part of the daily suffering that patients describe to their psychiatrists. The composition of the bacteria, their metabolic activity determine to what extent in a health condition, the kilo, the microorganisms, and the mucosa cooperate with the system enteric nerve and how behaviors and feelings develop as a result of this. Bacteria can potentially transform everything that comes from food into nerve-acting molecules. It must be noted that it is not that people with nervous disorders also have digestive problems, but that microbiome disorders are partly the cause of nervous system diseases. The intense exchange of information between the brain, the intestine, and the microbiota lasts for twenty-four hours a day, whether we sleep or are awake. All this communication is not limited to coordinating our basic digestive functions but has an impact on our human experience, which includes how we feel, how we make our decisions, how we socialize and how much we eat. And if we listen carefully, this dialogue can lead us to optimal health.

As the prominent microbiome expert David Relman of the University of Stanford stated: "Human microbiome is an essential component of what it means to be human." In addition to their indispensable role in helping us to digest many components of our diet, it is becoming evident that intestinal microbes exert a considerable and unexpected influence on appetite control systems and emotional operating systems of the brain and even on our mind.

Humans have a very peculiar part of the brain, namely the prefrontal cortex, which gives us the ability to bypass the function of altered brain circuits and learn new behaviors, several therapies help us learn these new behaviors.

How the intestinal microbiota influences our behavior represents a great challenge for the future. Intestinal bacteria are receptive to messages sent from the brain in the form of neurotransmitters, but they can also influence brain activity through the production of substances that will act on our behavior, on the level of anxiety and stress and, more generally on our Welfare.

Some studies conducted on laboratory mice suggest that the way to react to external stimuli depends on the composition of the intestinal microbiota. To achieve this result, researchers from the team of Professor Collins of Hamilton University, Hamilton, exchanged intestinal bacteria between two mice. The former descended from a group with a timid and anxious profile, while the latter belonged to a stock of "exploratory" behavior.

After the intestinal microbiota of each of the two mice was injected into the intestine of the other, the researchers found a change in personality traits and, consequently, in the behavior of both guinea pigs. The shy little mouse showed an adventurer behavior and vice versa!

The different bacterial strains that make up the microbiota would, therefore, affect what we are and how we act. We must begin to see the whole of our intestinal microorganisms such as the park ranger that helps us maintain biodiversity in a complex ecosystem.

One of the first indications of the possible influence of intestinal microbes on our emotions comes from the experiments conducted at the Institut National de la Recherché Agronomique (inra) on so-called germ-free mice, and the majority of studies published on these microbes and the brain have done reliance on this approach.

Scientists select germ-free mice by giving them a cesarean section and immediately transfer them to spaces.

Isolates places, where air, food, and water are sterilized, once grown up in this barren world, researchers study their behavior and their biology. The behaviors or biochemistry of the brain that are different between the two groups of animals can, therefore, be considered dependent on the normal intestinal microbiota.

Germ-free mice are less sensitive to pain and less friendly in interaction with their peers. Furthermore, the biochemical and molecular mechanisms in the brain and intestines are modified compared to those of normal mice; for example, germ-free mice showed less anxious behaviors than normally bred animals.

But when a germ-free mice were exposed to the intestinal microbiome in the first period of life, they showed none of these biochemical abnormalities. It has been deduced that when the microbiota colonizes the intestine, it somehow initiates the biochemical signaling mechanisms in the brain that affect emotional behavior.

The bacteria present in our intestines would, therefore, help us to manage better anxiety and stress, conditions that risk damaging our mental health. It seems incredible that bacteria can manipulate our behaviors for the benefit of their proliferation and survival, yet it is precisely what happens! In a recent study conducted by the team of Professor John Cryan of University College Cork, in Ireland, it was found that a mouse devoid of intestinal microbiota showed a lower tendency to seek the company of its congeners. From this, it is possible to hypothesize that our degree of sociability is partly influenced by the bacteria that reside in our intestines, which, to guarantee proliferation, always have an interest in favoring contacts with people. If it makes us uncomfortable the idea that nature predominates over education, or that our personality is not our hard work but the product of our genes, what should we say about a character made up of bacteria that live in the intestine?

Mice without intestinal microbes are antisocial, preferring to spend their time alone instead of their kind. Where a mouse with a normal microbiota chooses to accommodate any new individual being placed in the cage, the germ-free mice are with those they already know. Neurotransmitters are not only produced by human cells. The microbiota has its role since it produces chemicals that act in the same way, stimulating the vagus nerve and communicating with the brain.

The microbes that produce these substances act as a vagus nerve stimulator, sending electrical impulses, and improving mood. Rather than looking for a single uniquely responsible species, Allen-Vercoe, using Robogut (robot intestine) uses a holistic approach and considers the intestinal microbiota an ecosystem similar to a rainforest.

Extracting any species from the rainforest and studying its behavior while alone in a cage will not reveal much of its true nature. This also applies to microbes, which are influenced by the presence of other microbes and the compounds they produce. The idea that the formation of our microbial community can be influenced by the people we meet and the places we go gives new meaning to the idea of mental and cultural openness.

A NEW INTERPRETATION OF EMOTIONS

Incredible as it may seem, our intestinal microbes are in an excellent position to influence our emotions, generating and modulating signals that the intestine returns to the brain. Therefore, what begins as an emotion in the brain affects the intestines and the signals generated by the microbes, and in turn, these signals are retransmitted to the brain by intensifying and sometimes prolonging the emotional state. Clinical experiments with specific probiotics and fecal microbial transplantation have begun to directly examine the relationship between the intestinal microbiome and behavioral abnormalities. The intestinal microbiota that populates the interface between the digestive system and the nervous system occupies a key position to connect our psychophysical wellbeing directly to what we eat and drink, and in turn relates our feelings and emotions to the elaboration of food. According to an international team led by UCLA researchers, emotions could be partially driven by an unlikely source: our intestinal bacteria. The bacteria that colonize our intestines can influence the architecture of the brain itself. Who would have thought that simply by transferring faecal balls containing intestinal microbiota from an "extrovert" mouse could change the behavior of a "shy" mouse making it more similar to that of the donor?

Or that a similar experiment transplanting feces and their microbes from an obese mouse with a huge appetite would have turned a lean mouse into an equally voracious animal? Or that the ingestion of yogurt enriched with probiotics for four weeks could reduce the brain reaction to negative emotional stimuli in healthy women?

The growing knowledge of an integrated microbiota-gut-brain system and its close relationship with the food we eat is revealing how the mind, the brain, the intestines, and its microbes interact. Modern neuroscientists such as Antonio Damasio and Bud Craig, have proposed anatomically based theories on body-brain circuits composed of both sensory and active elements, the old theories have been replaced by a unifying concept of how our emotions are generated and modulated.

Craig hypothesized that all emotions have two components in close connection: a sensory element (body sensations) and an active component (somatic reaction) the sensory component is an interoceptive image of the body formed in the insular cortex by a myriad of signals neurons from various parts of the body, including the digestive system. This image is always linked to an action; according to Craig, the purpose of every emotion is to keep the whole body in balance. For Damasio, information on the body's reactions to an emotional state is stored as unconscious and articulated memories of physical states, such as muscle tension, rapid pulse, or shortness of breath.

In the last decade, the exponential growth of our idea of intestinal microbiota and its interactions with the intestine and the brain has led to expanding those modern theories and the inclusion of the microbiota as a third essential component in an expanded theory of emotions.

Our basic emotional circuits, related to the brain, are largely determined by genetics, present at birth, and epigenetically modified throughout life. However, the full development of emotions and bodily reactions requires a long process of learning, which continues throughout life, through which we train and perfect the brain-gut-microbiome system. Our specific personal development, lifestyle, and eating habits develop our emotion-generating mechanism, creating a large database in the brain that stores highly personal information.

It follows that the intestinal microbiota plays a key role in this process, as it allows us to generate highly personalized patterns of emotions. It acts on our emotions, mainly through metabolites that it produces. There are about three million microbial genes in the intestine, 150 times more than in the human genome. And even more surprisingly, we humans differ very little from each other genetically, since we share more than 90% of our 68 genes, but the assortment of microbial genes in our intestine differs greatly, and of them, only 5% is shared between two human beings.

The intestinal microbiome adds an entirely new dimension of complexity and possibility to our emotion-generating cerebral-intestinal mechanism. Since the microbiota seems to play such a central role in how we perceive emotions, whatever changes its metabolic activity, including stress, nutrition, antibiotics, and probiotics, can in principle modulate the development and reactivity of the circuits that generate emotions.

When it comes to something important, humans listen to their stomachs. Instinctive feelings and intuitions can be considered the two sides of the same coin. Intuition is a rapid and careful introspective capacity. Often you see and understand things suddenly without rational thoughts or deductions. You feel there is something unclear.

Instinctive feelings reflect a comprehensive and often deeply personal wisdom to which we have access. So what exactly is an instinctive feeling? What is its biological basis? And what role do the signals from the intestine have in your generation? When does an instinctive feeling become an emotional sensation?

In light of the latest publications by neuro-anatomist Bud Craig, there is the way the brain listens to the intestines and the microbes that inhabit it (and vice versa). There is increasing evidence that a constant flow of interoceptive information from the gut (which includes the constant chattering of the microbiota) can play a crucial role in generating instinctive feelings, thereby influencing our emotions.

Interestingly, while body movements are excluded, the axis of the Cerebro-intestinal microbiota is more active during sleep than at any other time. The powerful contractions and episodes of excessive secretion, which pass through our intestines every ninety minutes in the absence of food in the gastrointestinal tract, are fully activated during sleep, and during this period it significantly changes the environment for our intestinal microbes and their metabolic activity.

Similar gusts of reports from the intestine and from microbes to the brain, with all the neuroactive substances released during the process, I think may play a role in the affectivity that colors our dreams. Our entity is in a fluid balance, always committed to harmonizing stimuli coming from the mind and soul, from the environment and the body. The human being, in its entirety, is informed about the processes that take place in the intestine.

No "food" passes "unnoticed" through our body, the whole body eats. Food holds body and soul together.

➢ The precursor foods of neurotransmitters

• Tryptophan: Tryptophan is an essential amino acid; as such, it is essential for our body. Tryptophan cannot be synthesized by the human body. It is therefore important to take it with food or supplement it. The precursor of serotonin, melatonin, vitamin B3 niacin. It is also necessary for the production of many proteins. Starting from plant sources, we find it in legumes, including soy and its derivatives, in oilseeds such as pumpkin seeds and sesame seeds, in spirulina algae, in wheat germ, in dark chocolate.

As far as animal products are concerned, we can take into consideration cheeses, yogurt, fish, meat, and eggs. Metabolism of tryptophan could play a central role in the microbiota-intestine-brain axis. In the absence of the metabolic pathways necessary to synthesize tryptophan, it must be provided by the diet.

Most of the dietary tryptophan is absorbed into the small intestine through large neutral amino acid transporters and enters the portal circulation to be metabolized in the liver. Tryptophan is metabolized by the intestinal microbiota in a variety of compounds including indole that has been associated with cardiovascular disease. Although the role of tryptophan metabolites in microbiota-induced signaling is plausible, it cannot be excluded that the primary effect of microbial activity is the induction of a decrease in plasma tryptophan concentration. This reduction can affect serotonin and melatonin synthesis in the brain and thus secondarily influence brain physiology.

• Omega 3, group B vitamins, magnesium: the substances of good mood, some micronutrients play a vital role for the balance of the nervous system and our mental health such as omega 3 fatty acids (DHA), B vitamins and magnesium. The brain is the organ richest in fats after adipose tissue, and it is composed of 70% of fat necessary for the functioning of its cells.

The membranes of brain cells are made up of fat. Memory, concentration, and good humor depend on correct fat intake. Omega 3 are structural components of nerve cells, but also provide nourishment to "good" intestinal bacteria. By rebalancing the intestinal microbiota, they contribute to the anti-inflammatory action carried out by the "friendly" bacteria that produce not only serotonin but also other molecules able to counteract inflammation. They thus help restore the impermeability of the intestinal mucosa, thus preventing the passage of harmful toxins. The sources of Omega 3:

• Fatty fish like sardines, mackerel, herring, and anchovies, which have the advantage of being at the beginning of the food chain. They feed primarily on plankton and are not very heavy metals.

• Vegetable fats such as linseed oil, rapeseed oil and walnut oil to be chosen organic and cold pressed • Dried fruit and oilseeds such as walnuts, almonds, flax seeds, chia, and hemp.

• Vegetables such as Soncino and avocado

Chapter 10

FATTY ACIDS THAT ACT AGAINST THE INFLAMMATORY STRESS

Fish with a high omega3 content Fish / 100g Omega3 in mg Mackerel 2700;

Salmon 1800:

Herring 1700;

Tuna 1600;

Sardinian 1300.

Content of omega6 and omega3 in vegetable oils:

Vegetable oils / 100ml;

Thistle oil:

1 Oil of pips

2 Sunflower oil

3 Margarine (linoleic acid> 50%)

4 Sesame oil

5 Corn germ oil

6 Seed oil groundnut

7 Olive oil

8 Wheat germ oil

9 Soybean oil

10 Walnut oil

11 Hemp seed oil

12 Rapeseed oil.

Flax seeds: Walnuts, Macadamia nuts, Chestnuts, Sesame Pumpkin seeds, Sunflower seeds, Peanuts, and Coconuts.

Sources of B vitamins (B6, B9, B12) Veal liver, seafood, dried legumes, whole grains, spinach, watercress, Soncino, broccoli, wheat germ, brewer's yeast, green leafy vegetables Vitamin B9. For example, it allows the synthesis of neurotransmitters that are able to regulate mood As Naburo Muramoto says in his book the Physician of himself: "When the intestinal flora is luxuriant, it is able to digest the food entirely and to replenish the body with the necessary amount of vitamin B. An imbalance in the bacterial flora, derived from a non-assimilation of vitamin B, causes vitamin deficiency with symptoms such as ":

- Fatigue
- Pain in the body (especially in the legs)
- Tachycardia
- Difficulty breathing
- Mental confusion

Muramoto, recommends eating salads, one or two pieces per meal (especially those of rice bran), to increase the production of bacteria, to increase the intestinal flora, to obtain energy, wellness, and health.

Magnesium sources

- Green leafy vegetables, such as spinach, chard, chard, and herbs;
- Natural pumpkin seeds;
- Bean sprouts;
- Nuts such as almonds, hazelnuts, and walnuts;
- Bitter cocoa and extra dark chocolate;

- Legumes such as peas and beans;
- Whole grains
- Magnesium-rich waters

Chapter 11

RELEASE THE CHRONIC CONTRACTS THAT PREVENT VISCERAL EMOTIONS FROM BEING CARRIED OUT TO THE SURFACE, THE HARA MASSAGE

The abdominal cavity, in the eastern disciplines "hara" (source of life) contains many of the internal organs and extends from the rib cage to the pubis and the hip bones. The center of the hara, deep in the abdomen and our center of physical gravity, is a point on the midline of the front of the body, between the two hip bones. The hara massage consists of a specific standard practice which is part of Japanese medicine, whose origin was derived from traditional Chinese medicine. In reality, this practice is widespread in all traditional medicines, particularly in ancient Indian medicine.

This massage can also be indicated with the expression: visceral massage, indicating the direct action on the abdominal area. According to traditional oriental medicines in this area of the body, there are energy channels of great importance that can also be stimulated through the practice of massage.

Thus the action will not only refer to the organs of the abdomen and belly but the whole body. A quick result can be obtained when the subject is tense and accuses the contracted abdominal part. According to Chinese medicine, this happens because it is in the area of the abdomen that tensions accumulate.

Visceral massage gives excellent results in the case of constipation, irritable bowel syndrome with related symptoms (meteorism, spasms, etc.). In Eastern thought, Hara is the seat of human consciousness. It is the place where the spirit becomes matter and matter becomes spirit, in the continuous cycle of life. The hara contains our vitality, and its strength is an indication of how we can unify the body, mind, and spirit in our lives. From here come all our constitutional energy, our action, and our understanding.

It is the power behind the manifestation of our thoughts and dreams in the material world. Thus, a strong hara leads to the right action in the world. Since the hara is the real source of any health problem, small or large, according to the Eastern concept, an optimal state of health is maintained or regained by massaging this area. Conditions that do not yet manifest as a disease will not reach this point if you massage the abdomen for at least ten minutes a day.

This simple practice, if regular, can then intertwine with a balanced diet, exercise, and meditation to maintain the condition of well-being. It is also a very effective way to keep in touch with your body and improve your health, developing a healthy intellectual and emotional potential.

When the abdomen is modified, the mental patterns also change. Changes are transmitted to all levels of existence: physical, social, emotional, and psychological. The abdominal cavity contains various organs: large intestine, small intestine, liver, gall bladder, stomach, spleen, pancreas, bladder, and sexual organs. At the rear, the cavity is protected by the spine and pelvic bones. At the front, the internal organs are more exposed and easier to reach. They are protected by a large three-section muscle that extends along the entire length of the cavity. If the muscle is well toned, while remaining flexible, it will massage the internal organs when you do physical exercise, when you laugh or cry.

During the massage, vegetable oils are used, such as olive oil and sweet almond oil or specific oils, simple or compound, specially chosen for the disorder to be treated. The reference point of the massage is the navel around which circular maneuvers are performed clockwise with a constant and superficial pressure followed by deep pressures dictated by the detection of the contracted areas and by their level of contraction.

This massage has no contraindications except in the menstrual period and the case of intestinal colic in progress. In such circumstances, it must be suspended or implemented with specification

Competence. The abdomen, as a conformation and anatomical structure, is the softer part of the body. The softer, more flexible, the sweeter part. Let us treat it gently, gently. Let's take care of our tummy to take care of our visceral emotions.

To regain possession of our drive part and above all of the whole body without any dissociation. In Indian philosophy, the belly is expressed in the Second Chakra, represented by the Orange color, which is a symbol of harmony, creativity, and self-confidence. It is a symbol of awareness of one's abilities. To have confidence in oneself, one must regain possession of the body, of body sensations, emotions, and feelings without any dissociation.

This chakra is located on the abdomen, about three fingers below the navel. It has a name, Svadhisthana, which means sweetness. It is associated with parts of consciousness related to the area of pleasure, sexuality, the ability and willingness to generate, emotions, the relationship with food. This energy center represents the communication of our physical body with the spirit: the body informs us of what it needs and what it finds pleasant and desirable. In an ideal situation, we can implement this communication perfectly.

Chapter 12

WHAT WE CAN DO FOR THE HEALTH OF OUR MICROBIOME

"Observe: you have heaven and earth in you" Hildegarde von Bingen.

A GOOD MASTICATION CARE OF THE INTESTINE

How can we protect ourselves from the loss of vital mucus on the inside of the intestinal epithelium? We need healthy food, a daily supply of bacteria and food for them. And we need a food culture; very simply, for example, normal chewing! Already by chewing thoroughly, it can support the supply of bacteria. In the intake of food, the saliva of the mouth, secreted by the salivary glands, is the first supply channel with abundant quantities of substances that stimulate the mucus, also for the bacteria in the next digestive tract.

With an accurate chewing the salivary glands release about 1-1.5 ml of saliva a day and this one contains, among other things, various enzymes for the separation of starches, and also mucin. It can be understood how foods should naturally be mixed with saliva by observing a newborn that sucks quietly from the mother's breast.

Milk and saliva are mixed in a proportion of one to one because the child must process the food just slowly, and this stimulates the flow of saliva. Things are very different when drinking artificial milk from a bottle. Through a precise suction movement, the flow of saliva and the formation of mucin are stimulated, and starting from the beginning of life the team of digestive bacteria of the mucous tissues is abundantly stimulated to the activity and to be dense.

The fact that in weaning and the transition to artificial milk, the infant often suffers from diarrhea is also attributable to little intake of saliva and mucin and the consequent disturbance of microbial activity.

The microbiota in the oral cavity is also activated by the amount of saliva. If the mixture of food and sufficient salivary flow is lacking, it is likely that microbial communities harmful to the tooth enamel are multiplied here, as it is known from "bottle caries", which appear when the child is given herbal teas or sugary drinks at night, when the production of saliva is reduced, and the flow of saliva needed to digest the carbohydrates contained in them is missing.

If people are observed while they are eating, at the restaurant, in the canteen, on the street or the train, one almost gets the impression that this is an inevitable necessity that one wants to fulfill as quickly as possible.

Perhaps it depends on the fact that this food is often prepared without love or with unhealthy raw materials, so much so that one can hardly consider a food anymore and that, consequently, it is not even good. However, it can be observed that the bites disappear into the throat at such a speed that there is hardly any time to chew. The food is swallowed, and with the drink, on the other hand, it gets better. Who should take care of the bite chopping work? The stomach is a muscle with a soft mucosa and wrinkles and folds in it but does not contain teeth. Everything that is chewed too little in the mouth and is not mixed with saliva first subtracts itself from actually adequate digestion.

This has consequences for the whole subsequent digestive process, which is no longer mechanical but works mainly on an enzymatic level. When the food leaves the mouth in the direction of the esophagus, it should have the consistency of jelly, and when they leave the stomach, they should be creamy. Only in this case are they well assimilated.

For small seeds, grains, and sprouts that cannot be chewed thoroughly, it helps in practicing a pre-grinding. If freshly crushed in a mortar or more comfortably in a grinder, even sesame, linseed, sunflower or pumpkin seeds or spices like cumin, cloves, anise or coriander can be opened before the meal.

For older people with mastication problems, it is advisable to blend everything. Chewing thoroughly, therefore, we take care of our stomach and our intestines, but also of all the bacteria that live there. We try to keep our intestinal mucous layer unaltered which protects us from too great a permeability of the epithelial tissue of the intestine and consequently from diseases.

Chewing thoroughly keeps the detoxification processes moving. Some substances foreign to the body, such as alcohol or morphine, are separated especially through saliva (which is extracted from the blood plasma and released into the mouth by the salivary glands through their opening) and then they can then be expelled through the intestine.

It is interesting to note that in 2010 an endogenous endorphin, the opiorphine, was discovered in saliva, which has a pain-relieving and antidepressant power and is even stronger than morphine, without however having the side effects, such as intestinal obstruction. Perhaps long and accurate mastication will soon be applied as a complement or basis for psychotherapy in case of depression.

For several years the California doctors of the Santa Barbara Cottage Hospital have established that proper chewing helps after bowel operations. Doctors had prescribed post-operative chewing gum three times a day for an hour to chew gum without sugar and found that, after about sixty-three hours, this put the intestinal muscles back in motion, while in the control group, that he had not practiced intensive chewing, this happened only after more than eighty hours.

However, all this reinforces the importance of chewing. Our mucous membranes are therefore supported thanks to the activity of the glands that release the mucus. The quantities of mucus produced are stimulated by a part of the microbiome, that is, by bacteria that work in a team and simultaneously make sure that the cells of the intestinal mucosa also receive the necessary energy.

What if our digestive juices in saliva, stomach and small intestine are unable to digest, what we cannot use for the direct feeding of enterocytes, is exploited by the bacteria of our microbiome, and this happens in favor of the intestine and consequently of the whole organism.

By nature, food provides us with both of these components simultaneously: that which is directly digestible by digestive juices and that which can only be transformed by bacteria. Proteins, lipids, and carbohydrates are defined as "easy to digest" because they "pass" from the intestine to the blood via the first viable route.

Thanks to digestive juices they are directly split and broken down into small molecules that, through the enterocytes of the small intestine, pass into the blood and, through the flow of the portal vein, go towards the liver and other internal organs. And then there's the rest. Precisely because this remainder is not easy and immediate on-site digestion, it is transported to the large intestine and, here they are further digested and transformed by bacteria into compounds that perform tasks much more complicated than those of simple feeding.

FOUR NATUROPATHIC GUIDELINES

The challenge is rather to reinforce our "ground" to be subject to infections as little as possible, to strengthen the immune system, to develop vitality to the maximum, to allow the innate intelligence of the body to express itself in its full potential, still partly unknown.

Only in this way will we be able to live together in a symbiotic way with the bacteria that surround us and that we inhabit. The goal of naturopathy is precisely to optimize the individual "soil" and vitality to promote global health. Naturopathy derives from English nature, "nature" and "path," which means "path." Naturopathy is, therefore, the "path of nature."

This discipline allows individuals to follow the natural laws, which are also the physiological laws of the human body, to promote the vitality and the state of global health, and provides the body with the means to regenerate itself by letting its innate intelligence act. The return to a diet suited to our physiological needs represents today a fundamental point of which we are becoming increasingly aware.

By allowing us to provide our host intestine bacteria and nerve cells with all the elements they need to function well, nutrition is the first step on the path to wellness.

A diet adapted to our physiological needs and to those of the bacteria we host is the first indispensable step to be taken if we aspire to achieve a state of global well-being. However, other factors closely linked to personal lifestyles also affect the balance of the intestinal microbiota and our general state of health: pollution, the degree of a sedentary lifestyle, lack of sleep, physical and mental stress. So, to be happy, we try to know ourselves, to respect our profound nature, and provide our body with the means to guarantee optimal health at all levels.

1. REMOVE wrong foods (refined sugar, refined flours, and animal fats)

2. REPLACE the elements of an incorrect diet with truly nutritious foods and a correct lifestyle.

3. INOCULATE the intestinal microbiota with prebiotics, probiotics, and fermented foods

4. REPAIR OF THE bowel with substances such as L-glutamine, glycine, bone broth, colostrum, and phytotherapy.

Chapter 13

WHAT TO AVOID AND WHY, AND RECOMMENDATIONS

As we have seen, what we eat determines the type of bacteria we host in our body. If some foods promote the growth of beneficial bacteria that have a beneficial effect on mood, others cause the proliferation of harmful bacteria or even the destruction of "good" ones. The result does not change: deterioration of the intestinal ecosystem, dysbiosis with consequent impermeability of the intestinal mucosa, inflammation with negative repercussions on the brain, mood, and behavior.

Refined sugar

Pathogenic bacteria, yeasts, fungi, precancerous, and cancerous cells love refined sugar! Thanks to this food, they can increase in our body. This is the case of Candida albicans, which feeds on the refined sugar that we introduce with nutrition. Excessive growth of this microscopic fungus favors the permeability of the intestinal mucosa determining the passage in the blood of undesired molecules (the exorphins) that have an irritating effect on the brain. This phenomenon can manifest itself with personality disorders such as depression, irritability, mood swings, memory lapses, difficulty concentrating, or chronic fatigue.

Refined sugar is one of the worst scourges of our age. Some studies have shown that this food creates a dependency higher than that induced by cocaine.

A quantity that although far lower than that of the major consumers (United States, Brazil, Argentina), is still three times higher than that recommended by the World

Organization of Health. Refined sugar doesn't only promote the growth of harmful bacteria, but helps to increase the degree of acidity in the body, and it causes a rapid rise in blood sugar, fatigue in the pancreas and brain.

This is where the link between refined sugar and mood lies. Foods rich in refined sugars have a high glycemic index; this means that when we ingest them, the concentration of glucose in the blood (glycemia) undergoes a surge. The pancreas works at full speed and secretes insulin to regulate the entry of sugar into the cells, thus trying to maintain an acceptable amount in the blood. The sugar level then drops sharply: it is called reactive blood glucose. It is associated with a sense of anger, anxiety, stress, bad mood, fatigue, and a need for sugar that causes us to fall into a vicious circle that leads to dependence on white sugar. Natural sources of sugar are fruits, dried fruit, and whole meal bread, whole organic cane sugar such as panela or muscovado.

• Harmful fats, fats are essential for the proper functioning of the body, for the brain, memory, concentration, not to mention that the cell membrane is made up of fatty acids. It is therefore of vital importance to supply fats to the body, but they must be the right ones. Saturated fats, consumed in excessive quantities in our society, can promote inflammation, cardiovascular diseases, hypertension, or hypercholesterolemia. They are found in foods of animal origin (meat, salami, butter, cheese ...) but also in some products of vegetable origin (palm oil, copra oil ...). If consumed in excess, these saturated fats favor the growth of a putrefactive bacterial flora, with negative effects on the balance of the intestinal microbiota. But there is also something worse for our intestinal ecosystem: Tran's fatty acids. These are processed fats, hydrogenated, and used by the food industry to stabilize and preserve food.

• Refined flours; Today, unfortunately, a diet based mainly on this product is the main cause of malnutrition, constipation, fatigue, and numerous chronic diseases of which everyone suffers. If one thinks well of it, it is a fairly new product, the common bread in fact until recently existed exclusively in integral form. In the post-war period, the cultivation of wheat underwent profound changes following the mechanization and intensive agricultural cultivation.

The development of the society and the enrichment have led to genetic selection, which has favored the most productive and most suitable varieties for mechanization, such as wheat with a short stem (because it is less subject to atmospheric events). Often, from people, I receive answers like these: "I eat refined bread and pasta every day, and I feel great."

Of course, because the symptoms of "white flour poisoning" are devious, they are not revealed to our eyes so that we continue indiscriminately to consume it, not knowing that often many ailments or completely misleading ailments could be eliminated by canceling refined foods from our food. The bank flour once in the intestine forms a sticky and hardly disposable baby food, which if consumed occasionally does not cause damage, but if ingested daily and even several times a day it can lead to intestinal poisoning.

Sticking to the intestinal walls, it can reduce the absorption of other nutrients in the diet, and alter the microbiota with consequent changes in intestinal motility, stagnate in the intestine bringing putrefaction with abdominal swelling, pains, and smelly stools. In the colon, over time, they can become very thick incrustations and restrict the intestinal passage.

Whole meal flour, unlike the refined one although it is still a carbohydrate, being rich in fiber, is absorbed to a lesser extent (it has a lower glycemic index) and also reduces the absorption of fat during the meal, helping to eliminate it with the feces, cleaning the intestine and thus helping to stay in shape! There are approaches that anyone can try today without spending huge amounts of money becoming more aware of certain behaviors to cultivate, and help our microbiome in a natural and organic way

• We reduce the inflammatory potential of the intestinal microbiota by making better choices from a nutritional point of view (avoiding industrial foods and ready-to-eat foods, instead of increasing fiber consumption)

• We work as much as possible on our intestinal microbial diversity, varying the fiber intake

• Integration of medicinal mushrooms such as Shiitake and Cordyceps.

• We pay attention to prenatal nutrition and stress

• We reduce the amount of food.

• Regular aerobic exercise increases microbiota diversity

• We fast to starve our intestinal microbes (intermittent fasting)

• We avoid eating when we are stressed, angry or sad;

• We share meals with others;

• We learn to listen to our intuitive feelings;

• A good chewing cure the intestine;

IN PRACTICE, How to introduce the right amount of fiber into your diet:

• Consume a portion of raw and cooked vegetables at each meal

• Change protein sources by replacing animal proteins with vegetable proteins such as legumes at dinner.

• Consume a handful of oilseeds and dried fruit if you feel empty in the stomach mid-morning or afternoon

• Eat fresh raw fruit with the peel away from meals.

• Add to salads, raw or compound vegetables such as flax, chia, pumpkin and sunflower, and nuts such as almonds.

• Prefer whole grains or semi-whole grains to refined ones. If the microbiome is given a good diet, enough bacteria, an environment free of poisons, psychic satisfaction and an adequate rhythm of life, even an already ill intestine can be freed from its shock and return to a healthy entity as an organ of dialogue with mucous membranes and healthy rhythms, capable of promoting an adequate capacity for intake, digestion and release.

It is proven that the cellular junctions occluding between epithelial cells are reconstituted through probiotics, and their ability to open and close healthily is again restored.

A pulsating intestine according to a healthy rhythm, which has healthy cells and a sufficient microbial variety is essential for the general well-being. Experience teaches that as soon as the healthy flow of digestion and metabolism has been restored thanks to microorganisms, other stiffeners in the human being, be they psychic or physical, also disappear.

As human beings, we take a step backward from microbes, and we recognize the ability to restore health through the communication of all cells autonomously. The step of trusting the wisdom of microbes, who know on their own how a healthy coexistence can be lived, is perhaps difficult at the beginning and yet it can be liberating in many ways afterward.

We are not men we need to care for, but rather those beings who for billions of years, long before we existed, have forged this planet and above all made our life on Earth possible. Knowing this places us in a pearl of vital wisdom that is greater than us and on which, indeed, even new research on the microbiome, if we want to be honest, really knows very little about it. Bacteria are the real solution for existence.

In them, we can experience the transition between the visible and the invisible world. The way we treat microorganisms will decide in the future how human health will develop and if we will live healthier today. Not only does everything reside in our intestines, but also our hands, and perhaps even a little in our hearts. An important hallmark of human intestinal microbiota is its diversity and complexity of species. Several diseases have been associated with reduced diversity, which has led to a reduction in metabolic function. Studies have shown that it is enough to change eating habits to start improving the quality of the microbiota. The first changes are observed already from the first 24/48 hours; obviously, they are temporary changes that should be consolidated for changes that we can define as structural it takes at least 21 days, this is the minimum time to start consolidating a new macrobiotic structure. Once the microbiota has stabilized with the new eating and living habits, this new style must be maintained to make it increasingly stable and to be able to count on a powerful ally for our health.

FERMENTED IN DIFFERENT CULTURES

There are interesting fermented foods for their positive effect on the intestinal microbiota, and it is advisable to introduce them regularly in our diet:

• Olives in brine, in recent years some companies have resumed the tradition of sea water. If a solution of water and salt normally used for brine has 100% sodium chloride, in seawater we find only 60%, while the remaining 40% is composed of mineral salts. The analysis of this product has shown that in olives in seawater, there is an important presence of sodium, potassium, calcium, magnesium.

• SALADS, vegetables under water and salt Celery juice (Yin) can be used as a brine, since it contains natural sodium and maintains anaerobic vegetables, eliminating the need for sea salt, which prevents the growth of pathogenic bacteria. Here are some vegetables that are most widely applied: RED BEET, fermentation increases re-mineralizing and medicinal properties. The sedative is, therefore, suitable for evening meals for anxious people.

CABBAGE CAPPUCCIO Fermented is a panacea, very healthy, for liver insufficiencies, constipation, for rebalancing oily skin and acne.

CUCUMBER, A real treasure of water that fermented becomes a precious diuretic and rebalancing remedy.

ONIONS MEDICINAL FOODS, in the version enhanced by fermentation, it becomes an effective stimulant of all the body's functions, especially for the diabetic and the obese.

RAPPE, It is always "raped" consuming it cooked. Fermented is an excellent diuretic remedy suitable for gout and obesity. Consumed during periods of flu, cough, bronchitis, it also accelerates healing.

PUMPKIN, it is sedative, diuretic, and laxative. Fermented even more. • Sauerkraut - Easy to prepare at home, this type of cabbage is rich in fiber and vitamins A, C, K, and various B vitamins. It is also a good source of iron, manganese, copper, sodium, magnesium, and calcium. A 2016 study in the journal Functional Foods in Health and Disease concluded that two tablespoons (30 ml) of sauerkraut contain the recommended daily number of CFU (colony forming unit) of Lactobacillus. Based on these results, sauerkraut can be considered as a "probiotic superfood."

• Miso - This traditional Japanese pasta is made from fermented soybeans and cereals composed of millions of beneficial bacteria. It is rich in essential minerals, and it is a good source of various B vitamins, vitamins E, K, and folic acid

• Kimchi - spicier than sauerkraut, Kimchi is a dish of Korean origin, it is gotten by the process of salting and fermentation (which can last from one to several months) of kohlrabi and other vegetables (turnips, carrots, leeks, garlic, ginger, chili). It contains vitamins A, B1, B2 and C and minerals such as iron, calcium and selenium, the American journal Health has included it in the world ranking of the most powerful anticancer drugs.

• Umeboshi - plums macerated in salt, in Japan, at the time of the samurai, these salted plums were one of the most precious foods for soldiers, who ate them with rice and drinks as an antidote to battle fatigue and as a water purifier.

The umeboshi possesses remarkable medical properties, and they are rich in organic acids (citric acid and phosphoric acid) which help a rapid breakdown of harmful acids such as lactic acid and pyruvic acid, they sometimes present in excess in the body. Paradoxically, its high acidity has a strong alkalizing effect, and it can help maintain a healthy balance between acid and alkaline environment in situations such as fatigue, nausea of pregnancy, motion sickness or seasickness, nausea and stomach problems. Furthermore, it is believed to support liver functions and help the liver to process alcohol, making it an excellent natural cure for "hangovers."

• Tempeh - another version of fermented soybeans, it is a rich source of protein, a good choice for vegetarians. • Yogurt - Lactobacilli bacteria convert lactose sugar in milk into glucose and galactose, which further degrade into lactic acid, giving the yogurt its sour taste. Live bacteria remain in yogurt and make a valuable contribution to the microbiota.

• Rakfisk - salted and fermented trout for a period ranging from two months to a year) In Norway it is a specialty. In the typical restaurants of Oslo, it is served cut into slices to accompany boiled potatoes and raw onions and to be dipped in sour cream or mustard.

• Surströmming, from Sweden, is Baltic herring fermented for about two months and then preserved and canned in a light brine. It seems that the smell of this fish is not very tempting, but if one of the happiest people in the world is fond of it, they cannot be so terrible.

• Zha Cai, in the Chinese province of Sichuan, lactofermentated vegetables are an essential part of their culture and cuisine. Traditionally, when a child is born, her family will put the zha cai in a terracotta jar and continued each year until she got married, when she received the excitement as a gift. Twelve to fifteen jars indicated that the time had come. The zha cai is a ferment prepared by salting the green and swollen stems of a type of mustard, the Brassica juncea var tsatsai (sometimes it is considered a tuber, but it is a stem). They are full of bumps and makes them ferment, and the stem will be salted and pressed until it is dehydrated. Then it will be rubbed with chili paste and placed in a terracotta jar to ferment, even for years. Usually, it was rinsed before cooking.

Chapter 14

FERMENTED DRINKS:

KEFIR, this drink, of Caucasian origin, is obtained from the fermentation of milk made by some "positive" bacteria called Lactobacilli. Lactobacilli transform lactose into lactic acid, and thanks to this process, they multiply exponentially. Kefir in Turkish means "feeling good" and it is no coincidence that the drink we are talking about offers many health benefits:

• Anti-inflammatory activity

• Antimicrobial activity

• Antitumor activity

• Anti-cholesterol activity

Tryptophan is an essential amino acid abundant in Kefir, which has effects on the nervous system also because kefir contains bioavailable calcium and magnesium. The release of threonine, proline, and lysine is also sensitive. Kefir provides ample availability of phosphorus, which is one of the greatest constituents of our body and helps to utilize carbohydrates, and proteins for cell growth, for their maintenance and interactions, accumulation and energy availability.

Kefir is rich in Vitamin B9 (folic acid), B12 (cobalamin), B1 (thiamine) and vitamin K. It is an excellent source of biotin; these B vitamins help the body to assimilate other B vitamins such as B5 (pantothenic acid). The adequate supply of these vitamins acts positively in the regulation of the nervous system and the renal system, and they seem able to promote longevity. It is a good food product for lactose intolerant people because it is rich in Beta-galactosidase (lactase) and it is low in lactose because with fermentation it has been hydrolyzed about 30%.

KUM is an alternative to kefir as a drink. The only difference is that it is fermented with liquid yeasts. The milk is that of a mare, more sugary, which leads to greater alcohol content. There is not only Kefir and kumis as natural drinks with probiotic action. In the Turkish tradition, there are also other fermented products, such as the Shalgam juice obtained by fermenting black carrots, salt, turnips, baking yeast, and water. Fermentation takes place at 30 ° C for 24 hours.

KOMBUCHA Kombucha tea is a fermented beverage of oriental origin (Japan) has been known since 250 BC it is known as "elixir of immortal health" due to its extraordinary digestive properties. It is a sweetened black tea, fermented thanks to a solid macroscopic mass called "kombucha culture," a fungus that contains yeasts and bacteria (acetobacter) that produce acetic acid

- Facilitates digestion
- helps the work of the spleen
- Improves functionality hepatic

• Probiotic action for the intestine

According to some experts kombucha tea would have positive effects also on those who suffer from kidney stones.

REJUVELAC is considered a real elixir of youth. It is a fermented grain-based drink with a regenerating and therapeutic effect. Rejuvelac is also prepared with other ingredients: rice, barley, oats, rye, quinoa, millet. Rejuvelac also has the task of facilitating and regulating digestion, as well as strengthening the immune system by raising its defenses.

CHICA is a fermented beverage typical in Latin America and taken as a delicious aperitif. Chica is obtained from the fermentation of corn, cassava, or fresh fruit. The initial preparation involved chewing the corn and spitting it into an earthenware bowl; in this way, it was the saliva that triggered the fermentation. The method is still in vogue but replaced by the most modern fermentation techniques that gave rise to other variations of the drink: chicha kulli (produced with purple corn), chicha camba (for which peanuts and corn are mixed), willkaparu (yellow corn), and chicha de quinoa (with quinoa and black corn)

URWAGWA, Based on bananas and honey Ubuki, it is considered among the best in the whole Black Earth. The fermentation of this drink takes place in a wooden cistern covered with banana leaves. The juice that must ferment is obtained by mixing (or pressing) ripe bananas with the use of grass (inshinge) that often grows on the sides of the mountains. Subsequently, a preparation of water and malt of millet or sorghum (sprouted, lightly toasted and ground) called mulolo or mujimbi is spread over the juice, and then covered with banana leaves and stored in a warm place for three days.

The enzymes present in the millet or the sprouted sorghum allow the residual starch in bananas and malt to continue the fermentation process, which takes place thanks to the presence of the yeast (Saccharomyces cerevisiae) and the lactobacilli bacteria. In Burundi, the traditional national drink is the Insongo, the banana beer. In the heart of Africa, among verdant hills and deep lakes, the Burundians have decided to use bananas, the most common fruit, also to produce beer.

KVASS, it is a fermented cereal drink trendy in Ukraine and Russia, produced from malt, rye flour, and rye bread. It is one of the few examples of non-alcoholic cereal drinks (1.5-2 alcohol content); its taste is reminiscent of beer. It is a digestive tonic, it improves the health of the intestinal tract and strengthens the immune system, fights damage caused by free radicals, excellent for liver cleansing, and helps fight chronic fatigue, chemical sensitization, and allergies.

It contains and develops probiotics and digestive enzymes including: Lactobacillus casei Leuconostoc mesenteroides Lactobacillus reuteri Bifidobacterium

Saccharomyces cerevisiae Vitamins: A, C, K, B, folate Minerals: iron, calcium, magnesium, manganese, potassium Electrolytes, amino acids, antioxidants

PULQUE, it is an alcoholic beverage of Mesoamerica, widespread mainly in Mexico where, together with tequila, it is considered the national drink. It is obtained by fermenting the Salento agave juice and has alcohol content slightly higher than that of beer. In Aztec times it was used mainly by priests for ritual purposes and was considered a sacred drink.

TODDY Drink, it is widespread in Africa, in most of Asia, especially in the south, and in India, it comes from the processing of palm sap. Date palms, coconut palms, oil palms, carrots, or borage can be used. The juice is drawn directly from the wood: it is the contact with the air yeasts that immediately starts the fermentation. You get an alcohol content of 4%, for a naturally sweet and very refreshing drink. Longer fermentation can lead to a denser, more concentrated compound, and bitter counterpoint.

LASSI is an Ayurvedic drink made from yogurt, produced from sour milk, and the lassi was used for centuries as a yogurt drink before dinner. It is a popular product for getting probiotic bacteria.

MIRIN Less known than sake, it is another indispensable product of Japanese gastronomy, obtained from the fermentation of glutinous rice; this rice is steamed and then placed in contact with a specific yeast, koji. Depending on the alcohol level to be reached (Hon Mirin, the strongest, has a 14% alcohol content), fermentation has different durations. It is used mainly in the kitchen, to marinate rice and fish, to enrich soups.

REPAIR

In the REPAIR phase, special foods such as bone broth, gelatin, collagen, colostrum, L-glutamine, glycine, and Chinese herbs are included in the daily supplementation program. The scientific literature has shown that these foods can reconstitute the integrity of the intestinal lining, preventing large molecules of undigested food and "colino" metabolic waste, resuming the comparison with the colander, from the intestine to the bloodstream. The Chinese herbs that we are going to take during the repair phase depend on the type of diagnosis, it is usually defined by the examination of the wrist, the tongue, the situation of the intestine, the presence of inflammation, the tendency to be cold rather than warm, and from a further series of elements of Traditional Chinese Medicine.

Herbal formulations designed to "tone the spleen" and "excess dry moisture" contain active ingredients with healing properties for the intestine. For example, the combination of Sichuan pepper, dried ginger root, and ginseng root has been studied extensively in the treatment of Crohn's disease.

Easy recipe for the preparation of bone broth:

INGREDIENTS: 500 g of free-range chicken bones, 2 crow's feet (to thicken the broth), 1 carrot, 1 stalk of celery, a small onion, a handful of parsley, 3 cloves of garlic, a tablespoon of apple vinegar, a pinch of whole sea salt.

PREPARATION: put the bones in a pot suitable for prolonged cooking ("Slow Cooker," for example), cut the vegetables into small pieces and add them to the pot. Add the apple vinegar. Fill the pot with water until it reaches the filling line. Set to slow cooking and let it go for 18-24 hours. You can use this broth as a base for soups, soups or stews, or drink it as a hot drink.

Gummy blueberry gelatin candies

INGREDIENTS: 30 g of Grass Fed gelatin powder (from animals fed exclusively with grass), g of blueberries, 180 g of lemon juice, whole sugar, if you want to make them sweeter.

PREPARATION: mix the blueberries and lemon juice with a mixer. Pour the mixture into a saucepan and add the gelatin. Heat over low heat until a thick paste without lumps is obtained. Pour everything into silicone molds or on a ceramic plate. Put in the freezer until they have solidified.

Enjoy these snacks to nip the sweet cravings in the bud; these jellies will help repair the intestines, skin, and joints. Suddenly starting the intake of probiotics and fermented foods, continuing to feed on white bread, GMO and refined foods, and so on, can cause unpleasant side effects, such as abdominal bloating, the presence of gas, asthenia and mental confusion.

This is because probiotics feed the pathogenic bacteria that are already being depopulated in the intestine. It is first necessary to practice an elimination diet. Four weeks, or about 30 days, of the elimination diet, is a sufficient period to make these pathogenic bacteria die a little at a time. Only then can probiotic supplements and fermented foods be incorporated into the diet. I recommend introducing a fermented food every 3-4 days, in small increasing doses; monitor for no side effects such as gas, abdominal bloating, mental confusion, asthenia. Skip one day, or reduce the amount of fermented food until the symptoms subside.

Introduce one fermented food at a time, gradually increasing the dosage, and pay attention to the appearance of side effects. Many people report feeling an edge in energy and mood, but also in having obtained a beautiful skin and stone-proof digestion. Complete bowel washing is not a good cure for your microbiome. In this case, it massively intervenes on microbial cohabitation, with unpredictable results. A hydrocolontherapy is rather a wrong attempt to produce a clean solution.

Chapter 15

MEDICINAL, EXTRACTED PLANTS, WHICH ARE CONSOLIDATED (AND TRADITIONAL) IN THE TREATMENT OF THE MAIN INTESTINAL INFLAMMATORY FORMS

Aloe from Barbados leaves. The ingestion of Aloe vera can promote the cellular exchange of the gastrointestinal mucosa, through the support of tissue regeneration, as well as accelerating the healing of lesions or ulcers eventually present. Thanks to its magnesium lactate content, aloe vera is also able to improve digestion without causing diarrhea, it performs a compensating action in the normalization of pH, promotes a greater balance of gastrointestinal symbiotic bacteria. Alnus glutinosa (L.) Gaertn. -

Black alder gems, the gemmoderivato has anti-inflammatory properties on the digestive mucous, and it stimulates the adrenal cortex. It dominates the processes of post-inflammatory fibrinolysis and is active in all syndromes or inflammatory mucosal sequelae, whatever compromised tissue.

Cistus ladaniferum L. - Cisto gemme Il Cisto is a gemmoderivative of elective choice in the presence of neurovegetative dystonias, concomitant with marked anxious states, accompanied by fear and pessimism. The somatization of neuropsychic discomfort leads to symptoms related to the digestive system, even with intense and close spasms.

The intake of Cistus ladaniferum contributes to the reduction of the appearance of autoimmune diseases with a dystonic anergic component (gastritis, gastro-colitis).

Cuminum cyminum-

Cumin seeds, there is a notable efficacy in the use of Cumin at the level of the gastrointestinal system, it performs its functions of carminative, i., e. It facilitates the elimination of gas from the stomach and the intestine, thus allowing an easier digestive function. It is recommended, in fact, in the case of meteorism, especially postprandial and painful flatulence. In addition to these specific actions, Cuminum cyminum is recommended to stimulate the appetite, contribute to easier peristalsis, prevent intestinal fermentation and the ensuing headaches.

Eucalyptus globulus Labill.

- Eucalyptus globe-shaped flower buds, the plant extract from Eucalyptus meristematic tissues intervenes on the inflammatory phenomena of the mucous membranes, especially intestinal ones, and in the context of unbalanced sugar metabolism. Often, under these conditions, there is a chance of modifying the balance of the intestinal bacterial flora and the circulatory and trophic mechanisms.

Ficus Carica.

Fico gemme Ficus carica is an excellent glycerin macerate, known for maintaining homeostasis and psycho-biological rhythms, by its diencephalic, antimitotic, antispasmodic and sedative properties of the neurovegetative system, with regard, above all, to the cortical axis -ipofisario-hypothalamic.

These properties give rise to the excellent action of regularizing the rhythms of the gastroduodenal and intestinal activity, with regard to irritations, inefficient intestinal endocrine, colonic motility disorders, psychosomatic manifestations with spasmophilia, mainly at the gastrointestinal level, in the presence of , or not, of pyrexia, gastritis, dysphagia and duodenal ulcers.

Ficus Carica. - Fico radichette, the plant extract of Fico rootlets can reactivate the functions of the vegetative nervous system and the endocrine system in their relations with the CNS. It promotes the recovery of sensory awareness of physical functions and the possibility of their conscious control. It has mainly intestinal activity, influencing its motility, secretions, and absorption. This gemmoderivato is also a valid aid in overcoming dependencies on irritating laxatives and in preparing the organism for hydrocolontherapy and the use of probiotics.

Melissa officinalis L.

Melissa summit Melissa officinalis is mainly used as a sedative in anxiety states, with visceral somatizations and restlessness and also in the presence of dyspeptic gastrointestinal disorders of smooth muscles, thanks to its spasmolytic action. Useful, therefore, in the case of nervousness, hyperexcitement, difficulty falling asleep due to tiredness, dyspepsias, heart palpitations, dizziness, irritable colon associated with flatulence (carminative function).

Lime buds On the digestive tract this plant extract can be used validly in the treatment of various disorders, especially if on a psychosomatic basis such as gastralgia, dysphagia, bulimia, hypertonic biliary dyskinesia, pains of the primary dentition, gastrointestinal colic of the newborn, spastic colitis irritable bowel syndrome.

Ziziphus jujuba Mill.

Jujube young shoots, thanks to its antispasmodic properties, this plant extract is used in the treatment of dystonia with gastrointestinal spasms.

Artemisia dracunculus. - Drangoncello leaves and flowering tops the essential oil of Artemisia dracunculus, it can be used as a valid remedy, for the treatment of some disorders of the digestive system, as it can contribute to the improvement of intestinal function. The Tarragon, thanks to it is anti-inflammatory, antispasmodic, carminative, digestive, cordial, digestive, vermifuge, muscle and spasmophilic properties, it can improve digestion and intestinal absorption, as well as counteracting various disorders. In particular, this plant extract is particularly indicated for the treatment of dyspepsia, aerophagia, flatulence, singulation, intestinal spasms, inflammatory and spasmodic colitis, nervous dyspepsia, and slow digestion.

Furthermore, the aperitif properties of the active ingredients contained in the essential oil of Peppermint can stimulate food intake (contrast of in appetence and anorexia).

Juglans regiaL.

Walnut buds. The Walnut has an exciting organotropism for the lymphatic glands, the intestine, the mucous membranes, the skin, and the pancreas; furthermore, it promotes a structured antibody action thanks to the stimulation of Kupffer plasmacytes and macrophages. The Walnut could be defined as a precious pre-biotic, since this is its regularizing action on the bacterial flora even in the case of complex alteration of the relationship between fermentation and putrefaction in the respective intestinal compartments, for the normalization of diarrhea caused by the antibiotic therapy and in cases of abdominal meteorism, flatulence, intestinal distension of dysbiotic origin.

Magnolia Officinalis Rehd. Et Wilson Magnolia gems are useful in cases of impaired gastrointestinal motility and when there is a failure of symbiont microflora. It allows recovery of the bacterial flora that has been modified by enteritis or by taking antibiotics, and it can precede other rebalancing treatments. Often the alterations of the flora manifest themselves with nervousness, irritability, restlessness, and discomfort. Indicated in all cases of spastic gastritis, duodenal ulcer, meteorism, constipation, gastroenteritis, dysentery, flatulence, and dysbiosis with nervous disorders (irritability, hyperkinesia), localized pain and gastrointestinal inflammatory or infectious states.

Morus nigra.

Black mulberry buds. The tropism organ of the bud of Morus nigra is aimed both at the pancreatic/exocrine and endocrine function, as well as at the intestinal level, where it performs an interesting action in case of dysbiosis.

Ormenismixta.-

Camomile of Morocco. This plant extract is particularly indicated for the treatment of colic, intestinal disorders due to coliforms, intestinal parasitosis, and dyspepsia especially if it is with small hepatic insufficiency, biliary and pancreatic insufficiencies.

Zingiber Officinale. –

Ginger rhizome. It is beneficial for numerous disorders of the digestive system as it can: improve digestion; help restores optimal intestinal flora; to counteract the main disorders caused by dysfunctions of the digestive system. It can optimize digestion and intestinal absorption thanks to its properties that stimulate food intake (contrast of in appetence) and its ability to increase digestive and absorption functions.

It also has anti-inflammatory, antispasmodic, and carminative properties that justify its use in contrasting disorders such as nausea, diarrhea, constipation, colic, cramps, and flatulence. In the treatment of the main intestinal dismicrobial forms of dysbiosis, a type of fermentative type, that is characterized by imbalances in the intestinal flora related to the distal segment of the small intestine and the proximal tract of the Crassus, where a strong increase of enteric saccharolytic microbial components occurs. Among these are the most representative organisms, towards which the essential oil of Ginger that has antimicrobial action, are bacteria belonging to the family of Enterobacteriaceae and fungi?

Chapter 17

ESSENTIAL OILS

Considering the high antimicrobial properties regarding some enterobacteria, fungi, and parasites, some essential oils are used in the treatment of different forms of alterations of the intestinal flora. They are considered effective broad-spectrum antibiotics.

The antibiotic properties allow the abnormal increase of disorders to be contained at an enteric level, favoring the restoration of optimal microbiological and physiological conditions.

- Lavandula angustifolia Mill. - Lavender Vera flowering tops

- Ocimum basilicum Benth. - Whole plant basil

- Origanum majorana L. - Whole plant marjoram

- Leptospermum scoparium J. R. et G. Forst. - Manuka leaves and young branches

- MenthaxpiperitaL. – Peppermint leaves and flowers

- Pelargonium graveolens L. – Geranium leaves

- Rosmarinus officinalis L. - Rosemary flowering tops

- Satureja Montana L. - Savory whole plant

- Syzygium aromaticum L. Merr. et Perry. - Carnation nails buds

- Thymus vulgaris L. ct. linaloliferum - Thymus with linoleum leaves and flowering tops

Aromatherapy-phytotherapic mixtures aimed at the preparation of natural remedies intended for the

treatment of the various forms of intestinal dismicrobies
Bitter orange syrup

- Bitter orange e. fluid 5 p.
- Bitter orange dye 10 p.
- Simple syrup Bitter herbal tea
- Absinthe plant 20 p.
- Centaurea greater 20 p. • Bitter orange peel 20 p.
- Grass-clover 10 p.
- Aromatic calamus 10 p.
- Gentian root 10 p.
- Cinnamon bark 10 p. 97 Carminative herbal tea
- Mint leaves 25 p.
- Chamomile flowers 25 p.
- Aromatic rhizome calamus 25 p.
- Carvi (German cumin) bruised seeds 25 p. Colagoga herbal tea:
- Dandelion root 35 p.
- Chamomile flowers 25 p. • Mint leaves 20 p.
- Marrubio plant 20 p 98

"I was taught by excellent doctors and ignorant women to fear fever, scarlet fever, and the various diseases seriously called infectious. The clear and obvious fact is that there are no contagions and infections, but only conditions suitable to make people sick. The diseases are not classified in categories like dogs and cats.

The doctrine of specific diseases, enemy and contagious, is the refuge of the weak and fragile minds of medicine ". Florence Nightingale (1820-1910)" Is it not the continuous wrong living that leads people to get sick? Are not factors such as pure air and personal cleanliness, on the one hand, the stale air and intestinal dirt on the other, to make a difference, to determine the well-being or the sickness of people? Are not the diseases of natural reactions to the absurd and stressful conditions in which we put ourselves? "Florence Nightingale's lesson is more valid than ever.

CONCLUSIONS

According to the 1948 WHO Constitution, "health" was defined as a state of complete physical, social, and mental well-being, and not just the absence of disease or infirmity. For Chinese culture, staying healthy is a primary responsibility of the individual. It is believed that the strength of viruses, bacteria, and parasites can do nothing against those who, leave a healthy lifestyle, know how to keep in balance the components of his being and his defensive energy. The ancient medical texts affirm that there is nothing the doctor can do to heal a patient who has lost the desire to live and has renounced the search for the balance of his mind, mental, physical and spiritual. Thus the search for health cannot be separated from the search for happiness and inner harmony. Naturopathy and Western medicine can easily hold hands, even if they proceed on different tracks, have different languages, and see the disease differently.

Naturopathy could enrich the Western one by helping it to grasp the sense of disease, and the Western one could make holistic medicine more precise and scientific. Emotions, mental attitudes contribute to the well-being and malaise of our body. Diseases are the way the body tells us that we are going the wrong way, and we need to change our way of thinking, every illness is a lesson we need to learn.

Everyone inside us needs for success; each of us has a gift of wisdom. Our body as everything is the mirror of our convictions and our most intimate thoughts. I started this journey because I lived it on my skin, I didn't listen to body messages, then one day the body stopped me, and then I started to change my way of thinking concerning the past, concerning people and situations.

I started living here and now, and I discovered the pleasure of feeling myself, listening to my inner voice, my heart, and reconnecting with my most intimate part. The negative experiences of the past had moved me outside; fear, anger, disappointments deprived me of listening, I didn't trust my heart because I was afraid of being hurt. In the past, I gave more importance to the judgment of others, and I thought it was my thoughts that were different.

I understood that life is mine and that it is right to live it, and if others do not share my choices it is their problem. Thanks to this journey, I realized that what I consider essential for me is right; I learned to put my needs and my priorities in line. Fortunately, in the developed world, our health depends largely on the choices we make.

The human body, both inside and outside, forms a landscape composed of habitats as varied as those on land. Just as the ecosystems of our planet are populated by different species of plants and animals, so the habitats of the body host different communities of microbes. The microbes that we host, unlike the genes that our parents have given us or the infections to which the environment exposes us, we can as well shape them, cultivate them and look after them.

As adults, the food we eat, and the medications we take, determine our microbe's population. We treat them well, and they will return the favor. If we are planning to have children, we are responsible for their microbiome, especially if we are the mother. I am absolutely in favor of the choice. The choice is both a sign and a freedom enabler. The choice is the heart of civil society. And the choice gives individuals the power to improve their lives.

The choice made without knowing the information available does not make sense. The scientific research of recent years on the microbiota has revealed a new level of complexity and control of the human body and provides us with new knowledge on how our body, intended as a superorganism, is programmed to function.

The choices we make after being informed are our responsibility. The only thing I would like to suggest is that you make these choices carefully.

The microbiota is an organ of the human body, the forgotten organ, unseen, and it contributes to our health and our happiness just like the others. But unlike the other organs, this is not fixed. If the Genome Project Human has taught us something, it is that genes, nature, can predispose us to a whole set of pathologies, but if we then develop them or not it depends on lifestyle, nutrition, exposure.

In short, from our environment. Now we have a third actor: the microbiome is a strictly environmental force that operates on our possible characteristics, but it is genetic and is inherited. A good portion of the microbiome is not transmitted to the children through eggs and sperm, or even through human genes, but from the parents, especially from the mother.

Many parents hope to pass on to their children the best part of themselves, films like Gattaca imagine a future in which this desire is not left to attempt. Most parents also hope to offer their children the healthiest and happiest environment possible.

The microbiome, with its genetic influence but environmental control, gives parents the power to do both. In organic farming, agricultural and animal waste are composted, nutrients are replaced by large biomass proliferating microbes produced in the composting process. And in the same way in the human intestine, the nutrients that are eliminated from our body by the bowel movements are more than balanced by the healthy ecosystem that digests the raw materials, that is the food.

The intestine is an internal composting structure. The variety of foods provides many different nutrients that, in addition to feeding us directly, also stimulate the array of microorganisms in the intestine, each of which is in charge of removing a different food. Just like the compost, a real seething mass of microscopic life, it is the beating heart that supplies nutrients to a healthy biological garden, so our intestines are internal composts that nourish the body. Our body is like a vegetable garden that needs natural care to grow. This means avoiding the toxic chemicals from some food will be helpful. Today there is a lack of exposure to the great variety of microbes, and as a result, the immune system remains underdeveloped and compromised. In the biological garden, microbes are appreciated, put to work to recycle nutrients: they are like a flame in the ground.

Applying this approach to what we eat translates into a world of good health for us and the way to achieve this is, above all, the ingestion of fermented foods. Our health is based on the health of our intestinal ecology. For the naturopath, it is a priority to take care of intestinal health through the trillions of microbes that we inhabit. In the past and even today, it seems right that nature builds the health of its evolved children (plants, animals, humans) on the strong ecological health of its smaller creatures: fungi, yeasts, bacteria, micro-bacteria and other microorganisms that break down organic matter.

They are, after all, destiny and the source of all life. Shakespeare said all these centuries ago with the words of Fra Lorenzo in Romeo and Giulietta: "The earth, which is the mother of nature is also his grave, which is his grave is also his womb." As for me and my microbes, we are slowly rebuilding our relationship, now that I'm well again I know for sure one thing: my microbes take precedence. After all, I'm only 10 percent human. It seems logical that the healthy ecology of my microbes can benefit from my healthy-well-being.

Made in the USA
Monee, IL
30 January 2021